AF376209

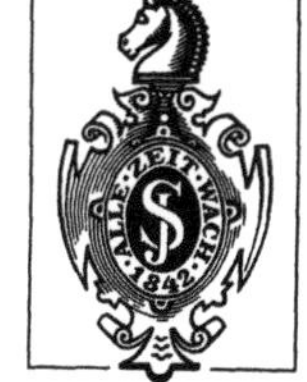

B. E. Strauer

Hypertensive Heart Disease

With 65 Figures and 19 Tables

Springer-Verlag
Berlin Heidelberg New York 1980

Professor Dr. med. Bodo-Eckehard Strauer
Department of Medicine
University of Munich
Marchioninistraße 15
D-8000 München 70, Federal Republic of Germany

Revised and expanded from the German edition:
„Das Hochdruckherz"
ISBN-13:978-3-642-67623-9

ISBN-13:978-3-642-67623-9   e-ISBN-13:978-3-642-67621-5
DOI: 10.1007/978-3-642-67621-5

Preface

In the Federal Republic of Germany today there are 6 to 8 million hypertensive patients. Of them, 3 to 4 million show organic cardiac manifestations of hypertension. Of all deaths occurring before the age of 65, 40% are attributable to hypertension, and the total mortality from hypertension is about 25%.

The high cardiac morbidity and mortality potential of the risk factor 'hypertension' lies in the development of cardiac hypertrophy, heart failure and coronary artery disease. In addition, hypertensive patients are predisposed to develop secondary cardiac diseases.

The aim of the present study was to analyse the myocardial function and coronary haemodynamics in essential hypertension, i.e. the most common type of pressure load imposed on the human heart. Consequently, the function and mode of operation of the hypertensive heart are described — a type of hypertrophy of the human heart which to date has almost been ignored in pathophysiology and diagnostics.

On the basis of the findings, conclusions are drawn for the differential diagnosis and therapy of the hypertensive heart accompanied by hypertrophy, heart failure and coronary artery disease.

This work was supported by Deutsche Forschungsgemeinschaft.

The support in translating this manuscript by Petra Fröschen, Christine Ebel and Cornelia Leisse is gratefully acknowledged.

Munich, April 1980 B. E. Strauer

Contents

Contents

1 Introduction

1.1 Rationale

Essential hypertension is the most common type of pressure load imposed on the left ventricle. Apart from cerebral, renal and peripheral arterial organic manifestations, it is one of the serious risk factors of coronary artery disease [44, 45, 116, 121, 122]. Both with and without concomitant coronary artery disease it will lead to cardiac hypertrophy, cardiac dilatation and heart failure. Effective treatment of essential hypertension is thus tantamount to effective prevention and therapy of hypertensive cardiac and non-cardiac organic manifestations. In view of the many ways in which the heart is involved in essential hypertension (coronary artery disease, hypertrophy, dilatation, heart failure), the detection and control of hypertensive heart disease are of particular importance. Although numerous findings are available today from investigations into peripheral haemodynamics, there exist hardly any measurements of cardiac and coronary parameters in essential hypertension. Therefore a long-term investigation series was initiated to examine ventricular function and coronary haemodynamics in essential hypertension, the results of which are reported in this book.

The most important results from the numerous investigations into peripheral haemodynamics can be classified as changes related to heart rate, blood pressure, cardiac output, stroke volume and peripheral resistance [13, 59, 65, 82, 112]. In stages I–II (III) of hypertensive disease (WHO classification) the heart rate is usually increased. With physical activity the percentage increase in arterial blood pressure is mostly steeper in patients with advanced hypertension than in normotensives. Cardiac output increases in stage I and decreases in stage III. With exercise the increase in cardiac output is abnormally reduced. Stroke volume as the resultant of cardiac output and heart rate is normal in stage I, whereas it is mostly reduced in the more severe types of hypertension. Arterial peripheral resistance increases in the more severe types of hypertension. The arteriovenous oxygen difference remains normal in most cases. Thus the initial stage of essential hypertension shows a slight hypercirculation due to the increase in heart rate, with only moderately increased total peripheral resistance. With increasing severity of essential hypertension, however, there is a progressive increase in total peripheral resistance and a decrease in cardiac pumping function.

Semi-invasive studies have shown that in decompensated essential hypertension the end-diastolic pressure within the left ventricle may be considerably increased. Despite high left ventricular filling pressures, the end-diastolic volume index may remain within normal limits, whereas stroke volume and ejection fraction of the left ventricle are considerably reduced [15]. There are electrocardiographic changes in the electro-atriogram which show biphasic broadened negative as well as flattened or excessive P waves. Often these changes are present before the appearance of signs of ventricular hypertrophy and the onset of disturbances of repolarisation [25].

Invasive studies using heart catheterisation and measurements of coronary blood flow in elderly arterial hypertensives without cardiac decompensation revealed a normal cardiac index in moderate hypertension (Smithwick grades I and II) and a reduced cardiac index in more severe hypertension (Smithwick grades III and IV) [5, 78]. Total peripheral arterial resistance was increased in all hypertensives. Coronary blood flow of the left ventricle and myocardial oxygen consumption were slightly increased in the hypertensive patients, while there was a marked increase in coronary vascular resistance [5, 78].

Morphology of the hypertensive heart shows a compensatory growth of the myocardium which correlates with the degreee and duration of hypertension. According to the concept of Linzbach this growth may be considered harmonious up to a heart weight of about 500 g or a left ventricular weight of about 200–250 g. It is the result of a thickening and growth of the already present myofibrils and muscle fibres [56, 57]. Only with higher heart or ventricular weights, i.e. pathological stress-induced hypertrophy, may a real augmentation of muscle fibres begin. On gross examination a compensated stress-induced hypertrophy can be recognised by a thick ventricular wall, a small interior ventricular volume and an extended outflow tract, whereas in the decompensated stage large ventricles with high end-diastolic volumes and eccentric dilatation may be present.

Both on clinical (symptomatology, ECG changes) and morphological (oedema of cardiac muscle cells, swelling and disintegration of mitochondria) examination, the hypertrophic hypertensive heart particularly often shows manifest signs of coronary insufficiency, for which the following explanations have been given: (1) arrest of growth of the lumina of the aortic coronary ostia with progressive growth of myocardial coronary arteries and coronary artery ramification; (2) disproportion between the hypertrophic myocardial mass and its supplying coronary artery system; (3) early involvement of the small intramural arterioles [43, 46]; and (4) abnormal intramural pressure resulting in an increase in the myocardial component of coronary resistance. In about 50% of all 50-year-old hypertensives morphological signs of sclerosis can be found in the small intramural coronary arteries. In vivo measurements from systemic coronary angiographies of changes in myocardial perfusion as a function of the stage of disease, of myocardial oxygen consumption and of the regulatory capacity of the hypertensive heart are not yet available.

Results from investigations into peripheral haemodynamics, ventricular function, hypertrophy and coronary manifestations of essential hypertension show that the effects on ventricular function primarily depend on the degree of hypertension and the resulting left ventricular hypertrophy, i.e. the *myocardial factor*, but also on the development of a coronary artery disease, i.e. the *coronary factor*. Both factors may result in global and regional contraction disturbances (Fig. 1). Thus when evaluating ventricular function and coronary haemodynamics in essential hypertension the degree of ventricular hypertrophy and insufficiency as well as the presence of coronary artery stenosis resulting in regional wall contraction disorders must be taken into account.

The prevalence of either the myocardial or the coronary factor or a combination of both the myocardial and coronary organic manifestations entails different patterns of hypertrophy, ventricular geometry and coronary haemodynamics. Therefore, as a function of the degree and duration of essential hypertension and as a consequence of secondary cardiac diseases, constellations of findings are to be expected which are typical of the particular stage of disease. Moreover, it is conceivable that pharmacological or therapeutic interventions, particularly the application of beta-blockers and digitalis glycosides, may result in a change in ventricular dynamics as compared to those of the normotensive left ventricle. Taking morphological findings and follow-up observations of the hypertensive heart into account, the effects on ventricular dynamics and the coronary system can be summarised as follows:

1. Hypertrophy of the left ventricle in essential hypertension is accompanied by changes in wall thickness, muscle mass, end-diastolic pressure and volume.

This leads to changes in those factors of ventricular geometry which determine the degree of left ventricular hypertrophy [3, 23, 38–40, 96]. Due to differing interactions between these variables the left ventricular wall stress varies. Changes in wall stress in turn result in changes in ventricular function, so that the left ventricular function in the course of essential hypertension is determined by the degree of hypertrophy.

2. At the same time as left ventricular hypertrophy occurs, the ventricular mass begins to thicken, leading to a change in ventricular dimensions. As a function of the degree, duration and intensity of pressure load as well as of secondary coronary and myocardial diseases, the cardiac and ventricular size as determined by roentgenography may vary from a normal configuration to general heart dilatation. With

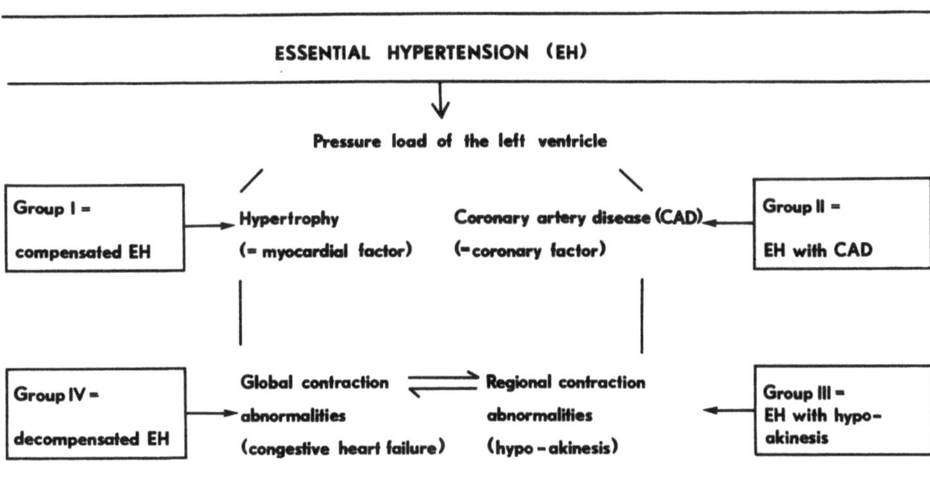

Fig. 1. Possible manifestations of essential hypertension on the basis of the patients examined. *CHD* coronary artery disease

identical absolute left ventricular muscle masses there may just as well be a left ventricle of normal size with normal or reduced intraventricular volume and a considerably thickened wall as there may be a considerably and generally enlarged ventricle with increased intraventricular volume and normal or only slightly increased wall thickness. Quantitatively similar mass increases of the left ventricle resulting from arterial pressure load may therefore, in essential hypertension, be accompanied by quite different ventricular dimensions. The ventricular dunction in turn is a function of absolute muscle mass, wall thickness, intraventricular pressure and volume or the radius. Any change in these parameters of ventricular geometry, e. g. following arterial and left ventricular pressure load in essential hypertension, will influence the ventricular function. Since these parameters change with the left ventricular pressure load they are also determinating factors of the degree of left ventricular hypertrophy. The degree of hypertrophy, which in these studies has been defined as the resultant of chronic left ventricular pressure load, with this resultant being dependent on such parameters of ventricular geometry as wall thickness, ventricular mass, intraventricular pressure and volume, is thus as decisive factor in left ventricular function.

3. In essential hypertension configuration and shape of the left ventricle, as well as the heart size as determined by X-ray examination, depend on the degree of hypertrophy and insufficiency, on coronary manifestations of hypertension (hypo-, a-, dyskinesis) and an concomitant secondary diseases [95, 96]. Consequently the heart size varies from a normal silhouette with concentric ventricular hypertrophy, increased wall thickness and normal or reduced interior volume to eccentric, generally enlarged heart silhouettes with increased interior volume and normal or thickened ventricular wall. In our laboratory observations occasionally indicated that in hypertensives ventriculography can show irregular hypertrophy of the ventricular wall distinct from qualitatively similar left ventricular hypertrophic states following cardiac pressure and volume loads [94, 96].

4. Arterial hypertension is one of the severe risk factors of coronary artery disease and leads to disturbances in regional and global myocardial blood flow and in the left ventricular coronary vascular reserve. Apart from being influenced by coronary manifestations of hypertension, i. e. concomitant coronary stenoses (*coronary factor*), it is conceivable that in essential hypertension coronary blood flow is influenced by ventricular hypertrophy and dilatation (*myocardial factor*). Few results are available on coronary heamodynamics in arterial hypertension [5, 78]. It has also not yet been determined whether chronic pressure load resulting from essential hypertension leads to a change in myocardial oxygen balance and whether ventricular geometry (hypertrophy, dilatation) may have a critical effect on myocardial oxygen supply.

5. Due to their positive inotropic effect, digitalis glycosides in the hypertensive heart are predominantly used in the treatment of manifest heart failure and the prevention and treatment of exertional insufficiency. Further to their use in these therapeutically objectifiable and clinically acceptable indications, digitalis glycosides are employed in the prophylactic therapy of the hypertensive heart with cardiac compensation in an attempt to delay the onset of exertional insufficiency. There are no studies demonstrating that such protective effect can be achieved by giving digitalis glycosides, nor is it known whether and to what extent coronary

blood flow and myocardial oxygen consumption in the hypertensive heart are influenced by digitalis glycosides.

6. In essential hypertension beta-adrenergic blocking agents are also used for the lowering of blood pressure [53, 68–70, 87, 110] and in the treatment of precordial pain or angina pectoris [6, 42, 53]. Due to their negative inotropic and chronotropic activity they are administered in an attempt to relieve the left ventricle and consequently to lower the myocardial oxygen demand, aiming at an improvement of myocardial oxygen supply. Studies on the relationships between ventricular function, coronary haemodynamics and myocardial oxygen consumption in essential hypertension under the influence of beta-adrenergic blocking agents have likewise not yet been reported.

7. Increased arterial vascular resistance may effectively be lowered by vasodilating agents, thereby lowering left ventricular impedance. For left ventricular overloading conditions, as in hypertensive heart disease, systolic unloading may be associated with an improvement in function. This may lead to augmentation of isovolumic and ejection phase indices in congestive essential hypertension and furthermore to recompensation of dilated and decompensated hypertensive heart disease. One preferably arterial and arteriolar vasodilating agent, hydralazine, has attracted special interest in arterial hypertension due to both its antihypertensive effect and its effects on ventricular function. Studies concerning the coronary and metabolic effects of hydralazine are not available. Moreover, the relationship between altered ventricular dynamics and left ventricular oxygen need under the influence of impedance reduction has not yet been investigated.

1.2 Aim and Scope

It was the aim of these studies *to analyse ventricular function* and coronary haemodynamics as a function of *pressure load* and the *degree of hypertrophy*, i. e. of the *quantifiable* cardiac *complications of hypertension* as determined by ventriculography, in establishing the *wall thickness* and *muscle mass*, the *mass-volume ratio* and the relationships between mass, volume and *wall stress*. Furthermore, systematic investigations are reported into the classification of essential hypertensives in view of diagnosis and prognosis as well as the therapeutic consequences that can be derived for hypertensive heart disease from the standpoint of the potential cardiac manifestations of essential hypertension. These studies involved the evaluation of patients with essential hypertension between 1969 and 1980 in whom cardiac catheterisation, coronary angiography, ventriculography, and reno-angiography were performed in order to clarify cardiac and/or non-cardiac complaints, symptoms and abnormal findings.

In detail the studies tried to answer and analyse the following questions:

1. What are the ventriculodynamic and haemodynamic characteristics of the hypertensive heart at rest and during exercise? Are there functional differences between the ventricular function in essential hypertension and that in other heart diseases accompanied by left ventricular hypertrophy?

2. What is the importance of ventricular hypertrophy in the hypertensive heart (myocardial factor) and of the coronary manifestations of essential hypertension

such as coronary stenosis and regional wall contraction disturbances (coronary factor) for the ventricular function at rest and during exercise?

3. How do coronary blood flow, coronary vascular resistance, myocardial oxygen extraction and oxygen consumption of the left ventricle behave in essential hypertension? Is the risk of ischaemia increased in the hypertensive heart with and without coronary artery disease, and can the risk of ischaemia be adequately assessed by examinations and influenced by drug therapy?

4. What is the importance of the coronary vascular reserve of the left ventricle as determined by pharmacology in diagnosing the coronary regulatory capacity in essential hypertension? What differences exist in comparison with the normal heart and the hypertrophic heart of other origin?

5. By what ventriculodynamic and haemodynamic factors is the left ventricular oxygen consumption determined in essential hypertension? What are the effects of ventricular geometry, degree of hypertrophy and ventricular wall stress on oxygen consumption?

6. What types of hypertrophy can be differentiated as a result and in the course of essential hypertension? Are there typical or specific types of left ventricular hypertrophy as a result of left ventricular pressure load due to essential hypertension?

7. How can the degree and proportionality of hypertrophy be quantified in essential hypertension and what are the factors influencing the degree of hypertrophy and left ventricular compliance?

8. What are the effects of digitalis glycosides (digoxin), of beta-adrenergic blocking agents (atenolol) and of afterload or impedance-reducing agents (hydralazine) on left ventricular function, coronary haemodynamics and oxygen consumption?

9. What diagnostic possibilities and therapeutic consequences can be derived from the examinations of ventricular dynamics, haemodynamics and pharmacology?

It must be noted here that essential hypertension is one of the most common diseases and actually the most common type of left ventricular pressure load. It should further be mentioned that systematic investigations have not yet been made into any of the problems mentioned above — with the exception of some single reports [13, 14, 26, 59, 73, 112, 116]. It is therefore the basic aim of this work to analyse for the first time the clinically relevant ventriculodynamic and metabolic changes occurring in the course of hypertrophy and development of a coronary artery disease in essential hypertension and to elaborate their implications for diagnosis and therapy.

2 Methods

The investigations on which the following reports are based involved a total of 158 patients with essential hypertension who for diagnostic purposes underwent cardiac catheterisation, ventriculography, coronary angiography and reno-angiography. Presence and degree of essential hypertension were defined according to the WHO criteria (WHO report [47, 121, 122]) after exclusion of all explicable and non-essential causes of hypertension. Cardio-invasive diagnostic procedures were only employed if required by the clinical condition or the need further to examine previous findings. In 73 patients these examinations served to verify or exclude the presence of coronary artery disease. Eighteen patients showed cardiomegaly. In 16 patients systolic heart murmurs possibly indicating organic lesions of the heart were found. A vitium cordis with haemodynamic implications could, however, be excluded in all cases. Eleven patients presented with cardiac arrhythmias not explained by their case histories. In 8 patients auscultation over the renal area revealed systolic murmurs. Non-essential causes of hypertension (renal, endocrine, cardiovascular etc.) were systematically excluded in all patients.

On average any pre-medication was discontinued 8–10 days before the invasive diagnostic procedure was performed. Over the same period the patients were strictly confined to bed when possible. There was no dietary regime. Where a hypokalaemia was present, oral potassium substitutes were given. Patients with diabetes mellitus and disorders of thyroid function were excluded from the trials.

The methodological details on the procedures used in cardiac catheterisation, ventriculography, coronary angiography, the determination of coronary blood flow and left ventricular coronary vascular reserve (argon method) have recently been reported elsewhere [9, 95, 96, 100–104, 106–109, 111]. All examinations were made in the morning after an overnight fast. The patients received local anaesthesia but no pre-medication. The catheters required were introduced by the technique of Seldinger [86]. Pressure measurements were obtained by means of Statham pressure transducers (P 23 Gb) or by simultaneous measurement using catheter-tip manometers. Cardiac output was determined by the thermodilution technique; the thermo-elements were placed in the abdominal aorta and the rectum (reference electrode).

The degree of left ventricular hypertrophy was quantified by measuring and determining its ventriculogeometric determinants from quantitative ventriculography and intraventricular pressure measurements. Left ventricular angiocardiograms were obtained before coronary angiography (Judkins technique) by intraventricular injection of 40–60 ml Urografin (76%, Contrac) at 30° RAO (right anterior oblique) [27–30, 41, 81]. The longitudinal axis of the left ventricle was directly determined from the ventriculogram, whereas the largest transverse axis was derived from the transverse axis running vertically to the bisected longitudinal axis. For each ventriculogram a specific enlargement and aberration factor was taken into account for evaluation and calculation of the volumes. Intraventricular pressure and volume were evaluated picture by picture in both the end-diastolic state and the systole until the continuously monitored circumferential wall stress of the left ventricle had reached its maximum. The peak wall stress (T_{syst}) was determined from the intraventricular pressure (P) (systolic pressure less end-diastolic pressure), the ventricular radius (r) and the thickness of the ventricular wall (d) according to the Laplace relation $(T = P \cdot r/2\,d)$ [3, 27–30, 41, 56, 79, 80, 99]. The interior left ventricular radius for each cinepicture was derived from the volume measurements $\left(r = \sqrt[3]{\dfrac{3V}{4\pi}} \right)$. Further, the thickness of the left ventricular wall was evaluated for each cinepicture in that the average wall thickness of an anterior wall segment about 4 cm in length extending from the equator 2 cm to each side was determined [30, 41, 75, 101]. It must be mentioned that the wall stress derived from the actively generated intraventricular pressure, the interior ventricular radius and the wall thickness represents an average value of wall stress related to the ventricular wall or ventricular thickness. This average value underrates the peak wall stress, which occurs in the subendocardial interior layer, and overrates the lowest stress within the ventricular wall, which arises in the exterior layers [38–40]. However, the endo-epicardial wall stress gradient is relatively constant in thick-walled systems and even in hypertrophic walls should not exceed 10%–15% compared to that arrived at in thin-walled model calculations [38, 39, 120]. Therefore no statements can be made as to the stress distribution within the left ventricular wall in thick-walled systems. However, the procedure applied permits useful measurements of the mean circumferential wall stress of the left ventricle. The value of ventriculographic determinations of left ventricular stress is limited by a potential quantitative overrating of systolic wall stress with very high degrees of systolic wall thickening and small intraventricular volumes as well as by a possible slight delay in the region of the peak systolic wall stress if the dissolution or cinefilm frequency is inadequate [84]. Thus under- and overratings of peak systolic wall stress are possible. In order to prevent a false evaluation of systolic wall stress in this study — in contrast to other procedures involving peak systolic pressure and end-diastolic volume [30, 41] — in each case those systolic ventricular dimensions (radius, wall thickness, volume) were considered which corresponded to the coincidental intraventricular pressures. On the other hand, all patients with dyskinesis, paradox pulsations and aneurysms of the left ventricle were excluded from the analysis since in those states considerable phase shifts of the systolic wall stress may occur. Thus potential false quantitative evaluations of systolic wall stress could be minimised. For determination of end-diastolic wall stress these limitations are less important.

Left ventricular muscle mass (LVMM) was exclusively calculated from the end-diastolic ventricular dimensions, i.e. from the measurements of end-diastolic volume and ventricular wall thickness at the time of the end-diastole [27, 29, 30, 38, 41, 75, 88]. These calculations were based on determinations of the ventricular wall volume including the specific weight of the heart muscle (LVMM = LVTV − EDV; LVTV, left ventricular total volume; EDV, end-diastolic volume). LVTV = 4/3·π·(L/2 + d) (M/2 + d)^2; LVMM = 4/3·π·(L/2 + d) (M/2 + d)^2 − EDV [30, 38, 41]. By this standardised procedure of determining ventricular mass used in our cardiac catheterisation laboratory normal values were found to be 90–98 g/m^2 body surface, whereas in extremely hypertrophic hearts left ventricular muscle masses of up to 400 g were determined. This is in good agreement with the ventricular weights as derived directly from anatomy [48].

Several compliance indices were determined for the evaluation or calculation of ventricular compliance [27–29, 33, 102, 103, 106]: as an index of volume compliance, the quotient of diastolic volume influx (dV) and diastolic left ventricular pressure rise (dP), which during that period run parallel, and in addition the quotient of dV/dP, normalised to the end-diastolic volume (dV/dP · V); as an index of ventricular stiffness; the quotient of dP and dV; as an index of the effective ventricular preload (ventricular end-diastolic fibre tension), the product of end-diastolic wall stress and (linear) muscle fibre stretch (volume distensibility) normalised to both ventricular wall thickness and end-diastolic volume, LMFS

$$= T_{diast} \left(\frac{dV \cdot d}{3 \cdot V \cdot dP} \right) [27–29].$$

Regional wall thickness, wall thickness changes and wall stress were determined in five ventricular wall segments. Perpendicular to the longitudinal axis of the left ventricle (connecting line between the middle of the aortic valve and the ventricular apex) five vertical axes were established at equal distances and the anterior hemiaxes drawn (Fig. 24). A tangent was drawn to the external ventricular contour in such a way that its perpendicular passed through the intersecting point of the hemiaxis and the interior ventricular contour, thus obtaining ventricular wall segments and distances of approximately centrifugal shape, when seen from a virtual ventricular centre. This technique was chosen since, in contrast to other techniques described in the literature, it helps prevent or reduce potential overratings of the regional wall thickness, particular in the basal and apical segments, which otherwise may occur due to distortions in the projections of the outer ventricular contours. The end-diastolic and end-systolic ventriculograms of all patients examined as well as each cine ventriculogram taken during the first half of the systole were evaluated picture by picture, until systolic wall stress, as continuously calculated from the intraventricular pressure and the ventricular dimensions, had achieved its maximum (T_{syst}). End-diastolic wall stress (T_{diast}) was derived from end-diastolic pressure and volume. Both parameters of wall stress were calculated on the basis of the Laplace relation. For evaluation of wall stress as a function of the regularity of hypertrophy, the maximal systolic wall stresses were determined regionally, i.e. in relation to the regional differences in wall thickness and in the radius of the ventricular wall segments M_1, M_2, M, M_3 and M_4. As further parameters of the degree of regional hypertrophy, the end-diastolic (d_{diast}) and maximal systolic (d_{syst}) wall thicknesses of the left ventricle as well as their percentage changes during systole compared to the end-diastolic initial values were determined in the five ventricular segments.

Left ventricular coronary blood flow was measured by the argon method in that argon was determined by gas chromatography in both arterial and coronary venous blood (coronary sinus) [8, 9, 93, 101, 109, 111]. To determine the left ventricular coronary vascular reserve, dipyridamole (0.5 mg/kg body weight) was administered intravenously over 8–10 min. The coronary vascular reserve was defined as the ratio between the coronary vascular resistance under control or resting conditions and the coronary vascular resistance during maximal coronary dilatation (dipyridamole) [9]. The coronary perfusion pressure was taken to be the mean diastolic aortic blood pressure less the left ventricular mean diastolic pressure. Left ventricular oxygen consumption (ml/min · 100 g) was determined as the product of coronary blood flow (ml/min · 100 g) and the arteriocoronary venous oxygen difference. Oxygen saturation in arterial and coronary venous blood was determined by Co-oximetry.

The left ventricular end-diastolic pressure was measured at the end of the atrial contraction immediately before the isovolumetric part of the ventricular pressure curve begins to rise steeply. The exterior or pressure-volume performance of the left ventricle was determined as the product of mean systolic aortic blood pressure and the cardiac index. The tension-time index was also determined by approximation in that pressure-frequency product was computed from the mean systolic aortic blood pressure and the heart rate.

Since arterial blood pressure, even under hospitalisation and heart catheterisation, may vary considerably [2, 52], in all cases those blood pressure levels were taken which had been measured simultaneously with the determination of the left ventricular volume. Thus the precondition was met that in all cases the actual blood pressure present at the times of measurement was taken both as a parameter of left ventricular pressure load and as a parameter for computing wall stresses. Thereby false interpretations of the relationships between systolic pressure, systolic wall stress and the mass-volume ratio were prevented in cases where the blood pressure rose under the conditions of cardiac catheterisation.

The comparability of the clinical correlations as determined under the conditions of chronic pressure load in essential hypertension with corresponding functional parameters of the left ventricle during acute changes in pressure and volume were examined in 98 experiments involving normotensive (NR) and spontaneously hypertensive rats (SHR) (Fig. 47). The parameters required (wall thickness, intraventricular volume etc.) could directly be measured during the experiments so that it was possible to make a qualitative comparison between the ventriculogeometric data to patients and the directly measured ventriculogeometric parameters in the experiment.

The findings obtained from the patient groups with essential hypertension were compared with those from the following patient groups (n = 484):

n = 12 Normal subjects; no hypertension, no hypertrophy, no vitia and no coronary artery stenoses
n = 38 Coronary artery disease; left coronary artery stenoses > 75%
n = 12 Hypertrophic obstructive cardiomyopathy
n = 22 Combined aortic valve lesions
n = 400 Patient groups with left ventricular pressure and volume loads associated with congenital or acquired heart anomalies [95].

The statistical evaluation was based on the mean values and standard deviations. The significance levels of the haemodynamic, coronary, ventriculogeometric and ventriculodynamic changes and findings were examined by means of the t-test. For the non-linear relationships between the mass-volume ratio and the

end-diastolic and maximal systolic wall stress values of the left ventricle non-linear
regressions were made according to a polynomial fit of second and third order. For
the pharmacological studies the mean values before and after the individual
intervention (digoxin, atenolol, hydralazine) as well as the mean values of the paired
differences were determined; the significance levels were computed on the basis of
the t-test for paired differences.

3 Results and Discussion

3.1 Ventricular Function at Rest and During Exercise

The examinations described in the present study were performed on a total of 88 patients who for diagnostic purposes underwent cardiac catheterisation, coronary angiography and ventriculography (Table 1). All patients examined had essential hypertension which was compensated in 76 cases and decompensated in 12. Of the patients with compensated hypertension, 32 presented with significant stenoses in the region of the left coronary artery (degree of stenosis > 75%). In 29, hypertension was associated with hypo- and akinesis involving more than 30% of the left ventricular hemicircumference. Hypertensives with left ventricular dyskinesis as evidenced by ventriculography were not included due to the abnormal temporal position of the peak systolic wall stress developed during the systole. The hypertensives examined were grouped and classified according to their degree of hypertrophy, their coronary manifestations and their degree of left ventricular performance (Fig. 1):

Group I: compensated essential hypertension without coronary stenoses
Group II: compensated essential hypertension with coronary stenoses
Group III: essential hypertension with regional wall contraction disturbances
Group IV: decompensated essential hypertension

Table 1. Case material (n = 88). EH, essential hypertension; CAD, coronary artery disease; LCA, left coronary artery

	Compensated EH	Compemsated EH with CHD ((LCA)>75%)	Compensated EH with hypo-akinesis	Decompensated EH
	n=15	n=32	n=29	n=12
Age (years)	44	41	39	49
Fundus of eye (47)	I/II	II	II/III	III/IV
WHO stage (122)	II	II	III	III
Duration of disease (years)	>8	>3	>8	>9
Angina pectoris	n= 8 (53%)	n=32 (100%)	n=26 (90%)	n= 3 (25%)
Previous myocardial infarction	n= 2 (13%)	n= 6 (19%)	n=23 (79%)	n= 3 (25%)
Cardiac hypertrophy (ECG, X-ray)	n=13 (87%)	n=27 (84%)	n=19 (66%)	n=12 (100%)
Cardiomegaly (X-ray)	n= 3 (20%)	n=11 (34%)	n=22 (76%)	n=12 (100%)
Abnormal heart murmurs	n= 9 (60%)	n=12 (38%)	n=13 (45%)	n=12 (100%)

The excercise tests were carried out in the lying position [4, 55, 82] using an ergometer load which caused the tension-time index as continuously computed to rise by an average of 60% compared to the respective initial values (about 1 W/kg body weight). Before and after the exercise tests the following parameters were determined: heart rate, cardiac output, aortic blood pressure, pressure within the left ventricle, maximum rate of pressure rise within the left ventricle and some derivative parameters.

The results of this study on the relationships between the end-diastolic volume and the ejection fraction of the left ventricle were compared with some recently reported measurements obtained from more than 400 patients with cardiac pressure and volume loads [95].

Results

Case Material. The patient groups examined (I–IV) showed no directed differences in age nor differences with respect to the duration of disease as determined from their case histories. Signs of left ventricular [89] and atrial hypertrophy [25, 26] and radiographic signs of hypertrophy of the left side of the heart were found in 20%–87% of the patients, in the three groups of compensated essential hypertensives with and without coronary artery disease, whereas they were present in 100% of the patients with decompensated hypertension (Table 1). The size of the left ventricle as verified by clinical examination increased with increasing coronary manifestations (coronary stenoses, hypo- and akinesis) of essential hypertension and was greatest in the decompensated hypertensives (100%). Abnormal heart murmurs were audible in 38%–60% of the compensated hypertensives and in all hypertensives with cardiac decompensation. The myocardial infarction rate was highest in those essential hypertensives with hypo-and akinesis (79%), and angina symptoms were found in almost all essential hypertensives with stenoses in the left coronary artery (degree of stenosis >75%) and with hypo- and akinesis (90%–100%). Corresponding to the severity criteria or the organic cardiac manifestations of essential hypertension [47, 121, 122] the clinical severity of essential hypertension was thus increasing in the following order: compensated essential hypertension (group I) − compensated essential hypertension with coronary stenoses in the left coronary artery (> 75%; group II) − compensated essential hypertension with regional wall contraction disturbances (hypo- and akinesis; group III) − decompensated essential hypertension (group IV). This classification of essential hypertensives according to their organic manifestations as verified by objective findings or quantified on diagnosis was taken as a basis for classification of the severity of cardiac involvement of all patients examined (Fig. 1).

Ventricular Mass and Dimensions. The mean arterial pressure in the essential hypertensives was increased by an average of about 50% compared to normal levels (Fig. 2). In groups I and II the ventricular mass was 40%–48% above normal levels while the figures for groups III and IV were 78% and 91% respectively. The ventricular mass per unit of pressure generated was considerably higher in groups III and IV, so that in advanced essential hypertension there was an over-

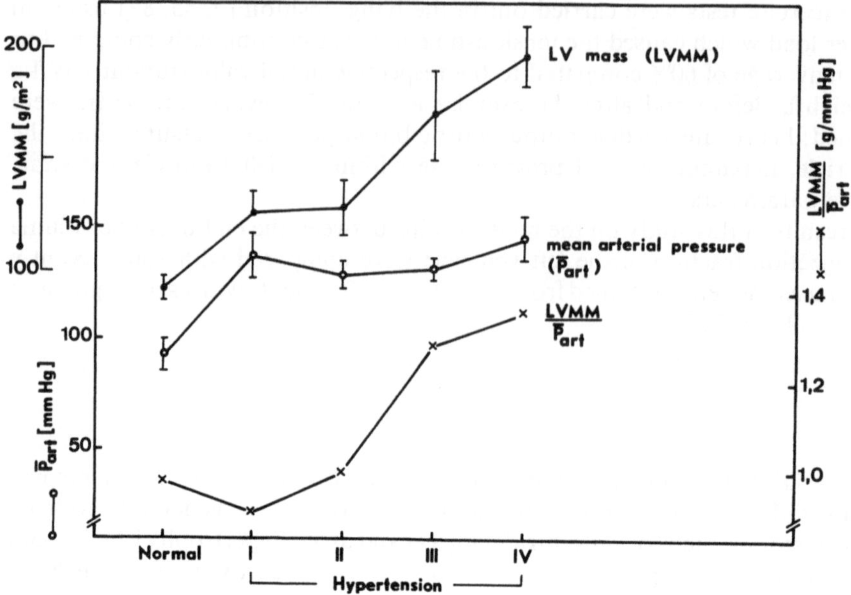

Fig. 2. Mean arterial pressure, left ventricular muscle mass and muscle mass per unit of pressure generated

proportional increase of mass in relation to the pressure load (mean arterial pressure) (Table 2).

The end-diastolic pressure and volume in all groups of hypertensives with coronary stenoses and regional as well as global contraction disturbances showed a marked increase (Fig. 3). The muscle mass, when related to the end-diastolic volume, i.e. the mass-volume ratio [23], was elevated in the compensated hypertensives (groups I–III) in favour of a considerable increase in mass per volume unit. In contrast, the mass-volume ratio in the decompensated hypertensives (group IV) showed a tendency to numerical normalisation, although only as a consequence of

Table 2. Mean arterial pressure ($\bar{P}_{art}$), left ventricular muscle mass (LVMM), quotient of left ventricular muscle mass and pressure generation, end-diastolic pressure within the left ventricle (P_{LVED}), end-diastolic volume (EDV) and quotient of left ventricular muscle mass and end-diastolic volume (mass-volume ratio) (LVMM/EDV)

	$\bar{P}_{art}$ [mm Hg]	LVMM [g/m^2]	LVMM/$\bar{P}_{art}$ [g/m$^2 \cdot$ mm Hg]	P_{LVED} [mm Hg]	EDV [ml/m^2]	LVMM/EDV [g/ml]
Normals	91±9	92± 6	1.01	10±1	81± 6	1.14
Group I	136±9°	122±11**	0.90	12±2	74± 6	1.65
Group II	128±6°	129±14°	1.01	15±4	80± 5	1.61
Group III	131±3°	168±16°	1.28	19±7*	112±16	1.50
Group IV	146±4°	192±15°	1.32	23±6**	147±17**	1.31

* p <0.05   ** p <0.01   ° p <0.005   ° p <0.001

14

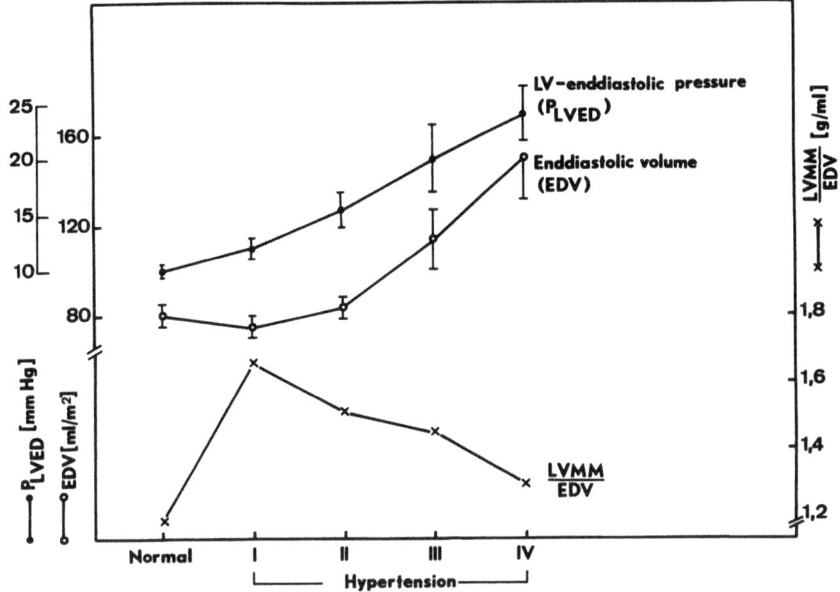

Fig. 3. End-diastolic pressure, end-diastolic volume and mass-volume ratio of the left ventricle

an over-proportional ventricular dilatation with progressively increasing mass. This means that in the course of essential hypertension at least two types of inadequate hypertrophy may occur: either an over-proportional increase in mass compared to the ventricle size, as in compensated hypertensives, or an inadequate mass increase not keeping pace with the progressively increasing ventricular dilatation, as in decompensated hypertensives.

Ventricular Function at Rest. Cardiac index, stroke index and ejection fraction were normal in the compensated hypertension groups I and II whereas they were considerably reduced in groups III and IV, showing wall contraction disturbances

Table 3. Ventricular function and contractility indices of the left ventricle. dp/dt_{max}, maximum rate of pressure rise within the left ventricle; MNSER, V_{CF}, ejection parameters normalised to ejection time; MNSER, mean normalised systolic ejection rate; V_{CF}, mean velocity of circumferential fibre shortening of the left ventricle; EF, ejection fraction

	dp/dt_{max} [mm Hg/s]	Cardiac index [l/min·m²]	EF [%]	MNSER [vol/s]	V_{CF} [circ/s]
Normals	1690± 90	3.82±0.09	72±2	2.52±0.18	1.62±0.13
Group I	2460±110°	3.95±0.08	78±5	2.68±0.21	1.71±0.12
Group II	2400± 94°	3.93±0.09	69±5	2.50±0.20	1.36±0.11
Group III	2310± 88°	3.22±0.10°	61±6*	1.98±0.38*	0.74±0.14°
Group IV	2190±102**	3.24±0.11°	40±8**	1.21±0.44**	0.44±0.14°

* p <0.05 ** p <0.01 ° p <0.005 ° p <0.001

15

and poor left ventricular function (Table 3). There was a pressure-dependent increase in the maximum rate of pressure rise within the left ventricle in all hypertension groups (Fig. 4).

The relationship between end-diastolic volume and ejection fraction [95, 96] shows that the ejection fraction of the left ventricle may remain normal even in severe arterial hypertension with left ventricular hypertrophy as long as there is no increase in the left ventricular volume (compensated essential hypertension with and without coronary artery disease) (Fig. 5). On the other hand a marked decrease in the ejection fraction is to be expected at the very beginning of ventricular dilatation according to the regression observed in patient groups with coronary artery disease and aortic stenosis. Thus essential hypertension, together with aortic stenosis and coronary artery disease, belongs to that category of heart diseases in which a progressive left ventricular enlargement is accompanied by a marked and grave reduction in pumping function and contractility as compared to that in other diseases of the heart or heart valves (mitral valve and aortic valve lesions, ventricular septal defects) and as measured by the change in left ventricular ejection fraction (Fig. 6). Comparable relationships were also seen to exist between the end-diastolic volume and the mean velocity of myocardial fibre shortening (V_{CF}) as well as the mean normalised systolic ejection rate (MNSER, [71], Fig. 7). Thus an increase in ventricle size as determined by ventriculography or X-ray is a suitable criterion for detecting a reduction in ventricular function in patients with essential hypertension.

Ventricular Function During Exercise. For the determination of the ventricular function during exercise two groups of compensated hypertensives of similar age showing different degrees of hypertrophy (group A: LV wall thickness, 0.69 cm/m^2; group B: LV wall thickness, 0.86 cm/m^2) and normal coronary angiograms were subjected to ergometer loads which caused the tension-time index to rise by an average of 60% compared to the respective initial values. With exercise the increase in the left ventricular end-diastolic pressure was normal in group A with moderate hypertrophy, whereas in group B with severe hypertrophy the pressure rose from 12 to 17 mm Hg (Fig. 8). The increase in the cardiac index in group A was higher than normal, while in group B it remained at 90% of the normal increase. The stroke index in all groups showed a similar increase. The increase in the maximum rate of pressure rise was normal in hypertension group A, whereas it was slightly reduced in group B (to 92% compared to normals, Fig. 9).

The relationships between the end-diastolic pressure and the cardiac index (Fig. 10) or the rate of pressure rise (Fig. 11) at rest and during exercise show a normal or increased reserve exercise capacity in group A with moderate left ventricular hypertrophy, whereas the hypertensives with severe left ventricular hypertrophy may at best show a slightly reduced reserve exercise capacity.

Discussion of the Results

The study of 88 patients with essential hypertension showed that the function of the non-dilated left ventricle was largely normal in essential hypertension, even with severe stress-induced hypertrophy at rest and during exercise. Contractility was not

16

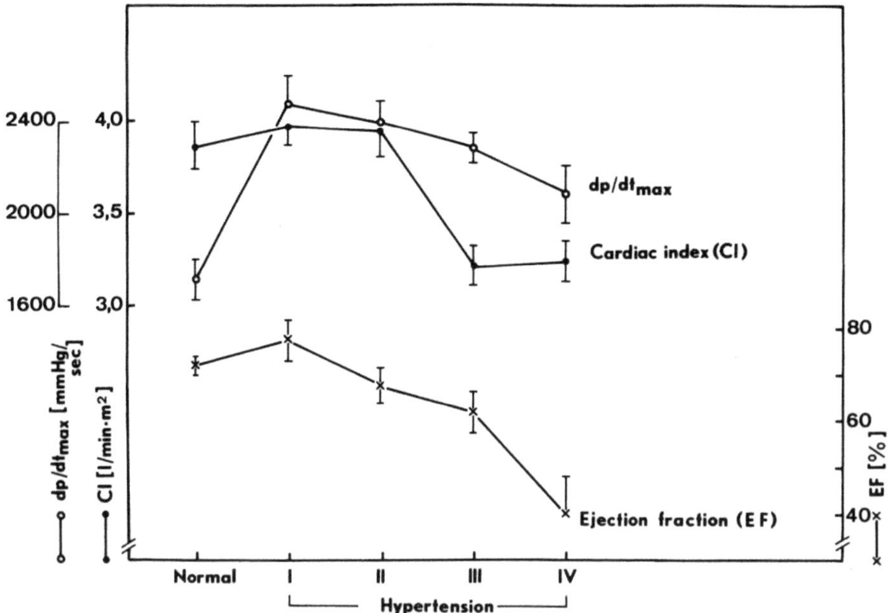

Fig. 4. Maximum rate of pressure rise, cardiac index and ejection fraction of the left ventricle

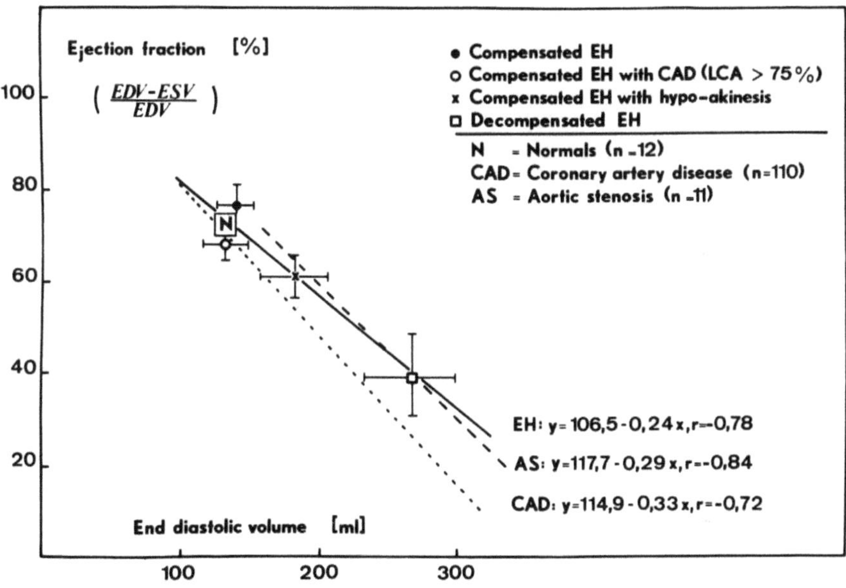

Fig. 5. Relationship between the end-diastolic volume and the ejection fraction of the left ventricle in essential hypertension (*EH*), coronary artery disease (*CAD*) and aortic stenosis (*AS*). Note the quantitatively similar slopes of the regression lines for the three patient groups. Further note the grave decrease in the left ventricular ejection fraction with increasing end-diastolic volume

17

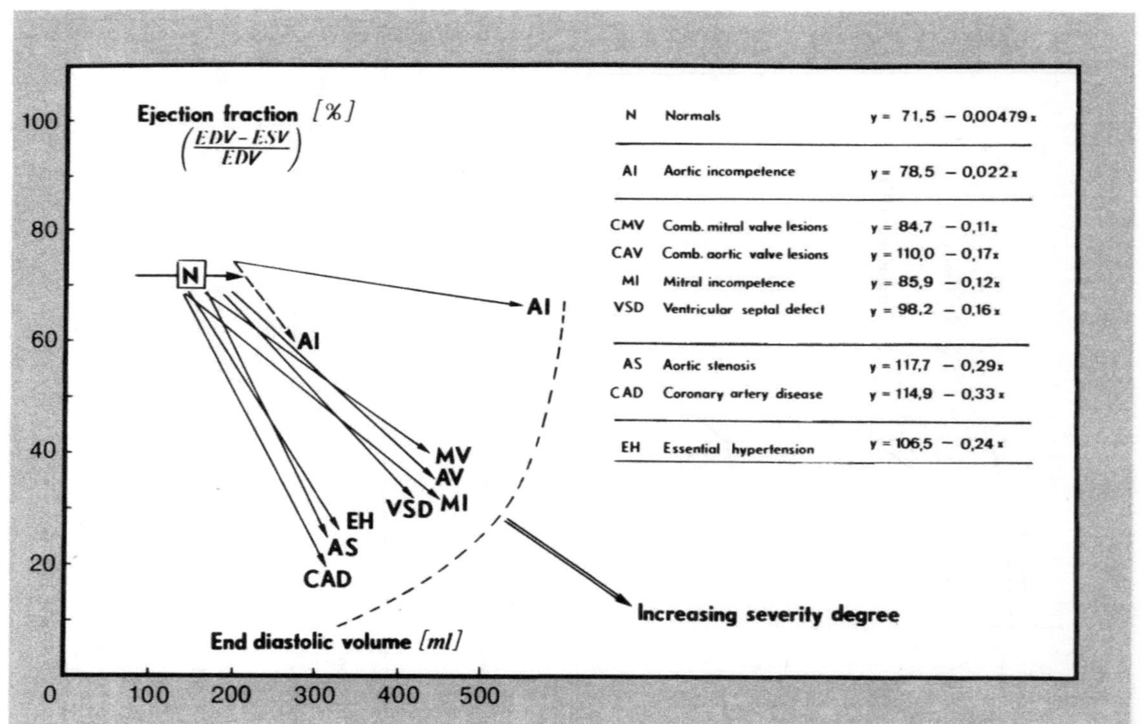

Fig. 6. Relationship between the end-diastolic volume and the left ventricular ejection fraction in patients with congenital or acquired heart disease. Note the considerably steeper decrease in the ejection fraction with increasing ventricle size in EH, AS and CAD than in patients with aortic and mitral valve lesions or ventricular septal defects (see also [95, 96])

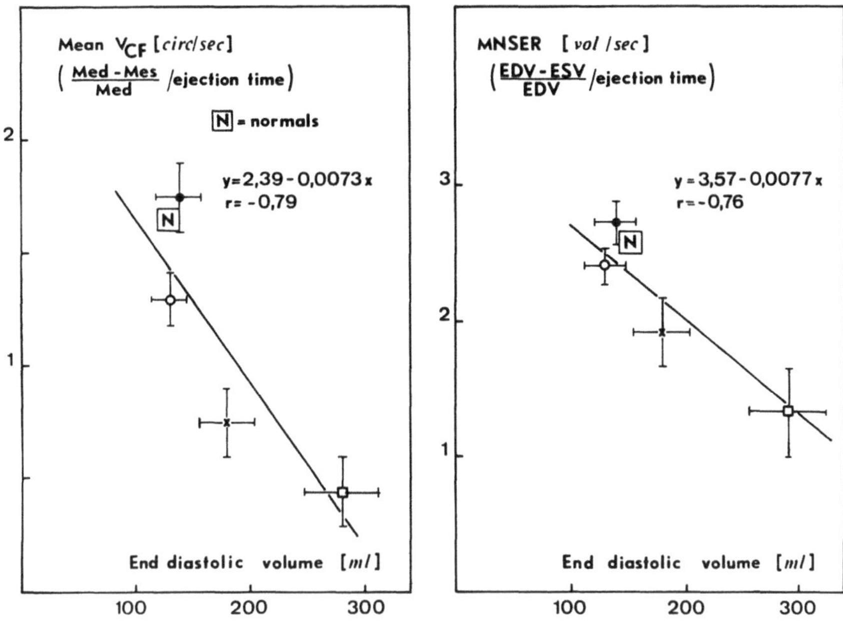

Fig. 7. Relationship between the end-diastolic volume and the mean velocity of circumferential fibre shortening or the mean normalised systolic ejection rate

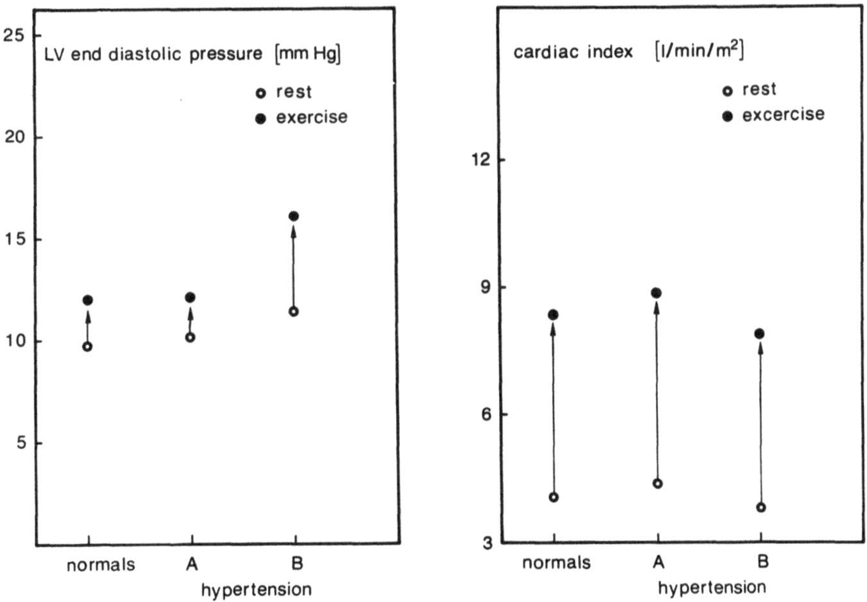

Fig. 8. End-diastolic pressure and cardiac index at rest and during exercise (n=14)

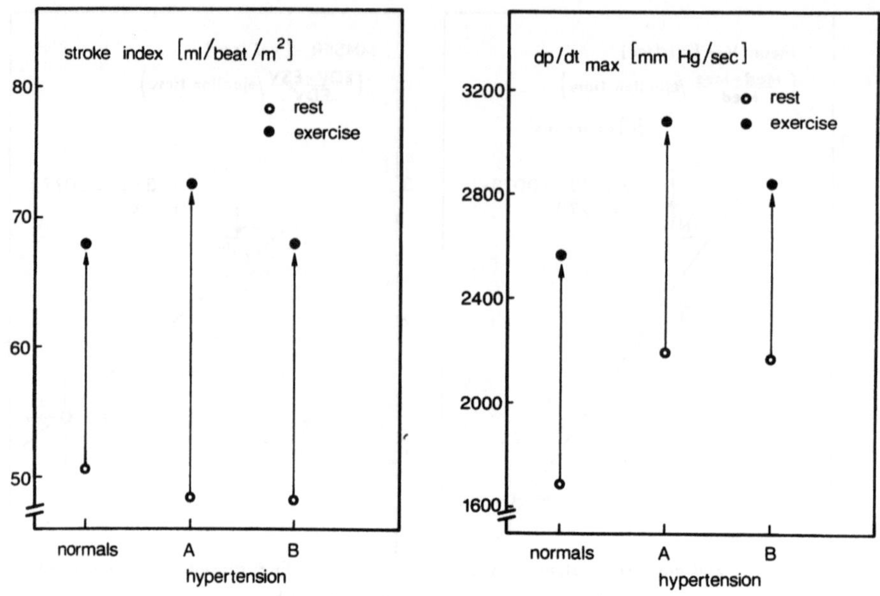

Fig. 9. Stroke index and maximum rate of pressure rise within the left ventricle at rest and during exercise (n = 14)

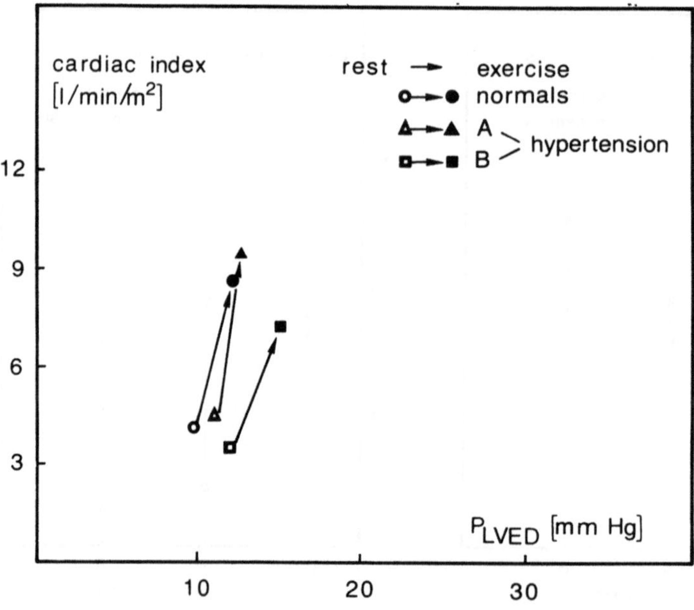

Fig. 10. Relationship between end-diastolic pressure and cardiac index at rest and during exercise (n = 14)

20

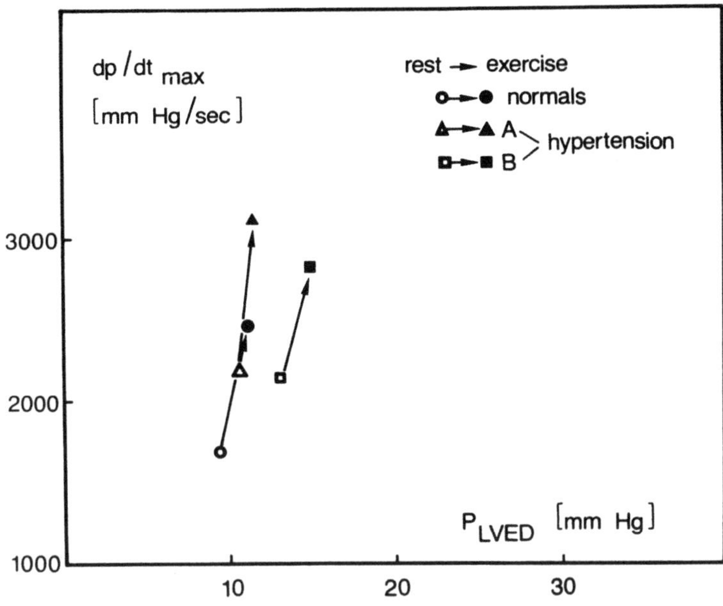

Fig. 11. Relationship between end-diastolic pressure and maximum rate of pressure rise at rest and during exercise (n = 14)

found to decrease. Reduced contractility may occur where ventricular hypertrophy (myocardial factor) is accompanied by coronary artery disease (coronary factor), where regional contraction disturbances are present and where there is a ventricular dilatation measurable by an increase in ventricle size.

The normal values obtained in hypertension groups I and II for cardiac index, ejection fraction, maximal rate of pressure rise and auxotonic velocity and ejection parameters (Table 3) show that despite a considerable degree of left ventricular hypertrophy with an increase in mass of 30%–40% (Table 2) there may be a normal or elevated ventricular function. This means that the stress-induced hypertrophy in compensated essential hypertension is not associated with a decrease in ventricular function. Thus the stress-induced hypertrophy in essential hypertension differs considerably from other types of stress-induced hypertrophy such as that following aortic or aortic isthmus stenosis where a significant increase in mass regularly appears to be associated with a decrease in ventricular function and contractility as early as in the compensated stage [71, 88, 91, 93, 107–109]. Thus no coincidence between an increase in left ventricular mass and a reduction in contractility can be shown to exist for stress-induced hypertrophy in essential hypertension. Apart from the experimental stress-induced types of hypertrophy such as that elicited by hyperthyroidism [93] as well as by Goldblatt hypertension [115], compensated essential hypertension in a patient therefore represents a clinical disease which differs from the concept of a reduction in contractility following a stress-induced ventricular hypertrophy. This may be due to the fact that the individual haemodynamic history, i.e. type, duration and degree of left ventricular pressure load, of patients with essential hypertension differs from the haemodynamic conditions of patients with other types of left ventricular pressure load. Thus it is not justified to assume that in general contractility is reduced following a stress-induced hypertrophy.

As shown by experiments employing graded levels of exercise, the reserve exercise capacity of the hypertrophied left ventricle is normal in compensated essential hypertension. This means that even during exercise the cardiac performance can be expected to be normal and that the presence of a significant degree of stress-induced hypertrophy need not imply that there is also an exertional insufficiency, which, however, will usually be present in secondary coronary diseases and more severe cardiac manifestations of hypertension (coronary stenoses affecting haemodynamics, regional wall contraction disturbances, ventricular dilatation). From this it may be concluded that measures of positive inotropic effect, such as digitalis glycosides, are not indicated in compensated essential hypertension with a view to improving ventricular function and contractility, since there is no impairment of the ventricular function at rest or during exercise which would justify their use. It has not yet been established whether the development of exertional insufficiency can be delayed in compensated essential hypertension by giving digitalis glycosides [64–66].

A clinically relevant impairment of the ventricular function and contractility may occur in essential hypertension where the following are present: (1) coronary stenoses (degree of stenosis > 75%) with or without previous myocardial infarction, (2) regional wall contraction disturbances (hypo- and akinesis) following coronary heart disease and (3) a left ventricular dilatation following coronary or non-coronary organic manifestations of essential hypertension. Since the coronary organic manifestations of essential hypertension are predominantly responsible for the development of ventricular dilatation, the reduction in ventricular function and the cardiac propensity to decompensation, the coronary factor, i.e. the coronary macro- or microangiopathy, is an important clinical factor of potential disease. However, hypertensives with a considerable degree of coronary stenosis may have a normal ventricular function even if they show a high degree of stress-induced hypertrophy, so that the sole existence of coronary stenoses does not necessarily limit ventricular function in the hypertensive patient. On the other hand, the following combinations in essential hypertension are nearly always tantamount to an established clinical impairment of the ventricular function:

1. Coronary stenosis and previous myocardial infarction,
2. Coronary stenosis and regional wall contraction disturbances,
3. Previous myocardial infarction and/or regional wall contraction disturbances even without the identification of coronary stenosis by coronary angiography.

Secondary coronary diseases seem to have a similar quantitative effect on left ventricular function and contractitilty in essential hypertension as they have in normotensive coronary artery disease.

The changes in ventricular function and contractility in essential hypertension clearly correlate with the size of the left ventricle as determined by ventriculography. With increasing ventricle size the ejection fraction and the ejection phase parameters that have been normalised with respect to time or velocity decrease.

Since the ejection fraction depends both on pre- and afterload and on contractility [85], it may be concluded that the ventricular function and contractility in essential hypertension decreases as the heart or ventricle size increases. This means that the ventricle size as determined by ventriculography or chest X-ray may be considered a useful clinical criterion for the evaluation of the ventricular function in essential hypertension. Since uncomplicated hypertension in itself does not represent an indication for ventriculography and thus for determination of the ventricle size by ventriculography, there is the logical consequence for clinical practice that it is possible approximately to evaluate the ventricular function and cardiac performance in essential hypertension by obtaining a standardised chest X-ray and determining the heart size or the size of the left ventricle.

A basis for evaluating the cardiac severity of essential hypertension as well as for the decision regarding which therapeutic measure to take is provided these determinations of heart and ventricle size, particularly if follow-up examinations are carried out. However, it must be kept in mind that the criterion of 'heart size' implies changes in the heart or ventricle size resulting from different causes. Thus cardiac enlargement in essential hypertension may, apart from other possible causes, result from ventricular hypertrophy without ventricular dilatation, from ventricular hypertrophy and dilatation or from regional wall contraction disturbances, particularly if accompanying coronary artery disease, or it may be a reflection of a global contraction disorder of the left ventricle in manifest insufficiency at rest or up on effort. The cause in almost all cases is the abnormal pressure load with its consequences of ventricular hypertrophy (myocardial factor) and coronary artery disease (coronary factor). It is therefore conceivable that an extended regional wall contraction disorder in essential hypertension with a resulting increase in the akinetic segment results in a similar quantitative increase in the ventricle size and decrease in the ejection fraction and ventricular function as does a hypertensive ventricular hypertrophy with ventricular dilatation but without coronary artery disease. The ejection fraction can be shown to decrease with increasing ventricular dilatation in both normotensive coronary artery disease and stress-induced left ventricular hypertrophy following aortic stenosis (Fig. 5). Likewise, there is an almost identical correlation between the end-diastolic volume and the ejection fraction in essential hypertension. Therefore it can be concluded that normotensive coronary artery disease, aortic stenosis without coronary artery disease and essential hypertension with and without coronary artery disease show a comparably severe decrease in the ejection fraction and ventricular function with increasing ventricle size and that the determination of the relationship between both variables meets the requirements for evaluating the contractility with respect to its function and its implications for therapy in these diseases.

3.2 Coronary Blood Flow, Coronary Reserve and Myocardial Oxygen Consumption

It is the purpose of this section to analyse (1) the coronary blood flow, coronary reserve and myocardial oxygen consumption in a larger sample of patients with essential hypertension, and (2) the influence of the coronary factor on the coronary functional parameters and the influence of the myocardial factor on the myocardial oxygen consumption by quantitative determination of the degree of hypertrophy, of ventricular dilatation and of the mass-volume ratio.

The investigations comprised

63 patients with essential hypertension
38 patients with coronary artery disease
12 patients with hypertrophic obstructive cardiomyopathy and
22 patients with aortic valve lesions

who for diagnostic purposes underwent cardiac catheterisation, ventriculography and coronary angiography. The indication to apply invasive diagnostic procedures was given by the clinical symptoms and the constellation of findings (Table 4).

For quantification of the degree of left ventricular hypertrophy, in addition to the ventricular dimensions (end-diastolic volume, end-systolic volume, wall thickness and muscle mass) the mass-volume ratio was determined according to the wall thickness-radius ratio [11, 12, 23]. The measurements of the wall thickness and the calculations of the ventricular mass were exclusively based on the end-diastolic ventricular dimensions. The parameter chosen for the afterload was the peak systolic wall stress of the left ventricle and it was calculated by correlating diagnostic images to the appropriate intraventricular pressures and wall thickness values.

Results

Case Material. In 42 of the 63 hypertensives examined (67%) coronary angiography revealed coronary stenoses of more than 75% in one main branch of the left coronary artery (Table 4). Twenty-one patients (33%) showed normal coronary angiograms of both the left and right coronary arteries; there were no wall contraction disturbances (hypo- and akinesis). Angina pectoris was clinically evident in all hypertensives with coronary artery disease and in 62% of the patients with essential hypertension without coronary artery disease. Fourteen (52%) of the patients had experienced previous myocardial infarctions. Signs of cardiac hypertrophy (ECG, chest X-ray) were found in 67 patients (74%). Abnormal heart murmurs were audible in 43 patients (38%).

Table 4. Case material. EH, essential hypertension; CAD, coronary artery disease

	EH without CHD (n = 21)	EH with CHD (n = 42)	CHD without EH (n = 38)
Age (years)	39	40	44
Optic fundus	II	II	–
WHO stage [122]	II	II/III	–
Duration of disease (yrs)	>6	>8	>4
Angina pectoris	n = 13 (62%)	n = 42 (100%)	n = 38 (100%)
Previous myocardial infarction	n = 3 (14%)	n = 22 (52%)	n = 16 (42%)
Cardiac hypertrophy (ECG, X-ray)	n = 14 (67%)	n = 31 (74%)	n = 2 (5%)
Abnormal heart murmurs	n = 9 (43%)	n = 16 (38%)	n = 12 (32%)

Coronary Blood Flow, Coronary Resistance and Coronary Reserve. Left ventricular coronary blood flow at rest in the entire group of hypertensives showed a mean increase of 16% compared to normal subjects (Fig. 12), whereas the coronary vascular resistance was increased by 38%. The mean increase in coronary perfusion pressure, i.e. the mean diastolic aortic blood pressure less the mean diastolic pressure within the left ventricle, was 56% (Fig. 13). The arteriocoronary venous oxygen difference was slightly elevated.

The coronary vascular reserve of the left ventricle as determined by pharmacological methods in compensated hypertensives without coronary artery disease remained at 72% of normal values, whereas it was reduced to 42% in compensated hypertensives with coronary artery disease (Fig. 14, Table 5). The coronary vascular reserves were thus similar in essential hypertension with coronary artery disease and in coronary artery disease without essential hypertension, so that the occurrence of the coronary factor in essential hypertension with respect to the coronary vascular reserve seems to indicate that the risk of ischaemia is at least qualitatively comparable to that in normotensive coronary artery disease.

It should be mentioned that the coronary vascular reserve was also considerably reduced in compensated essential hypertension without coronary artery disease, i.e. with normal coronary angiograms (Fig. 14). There was no relationship between the decrease in coronary vascular reserve and the end-diastolic pressure, nor between the end-diastolic volume and wall stress. However, the coronary vascular reserve was found to decrease with increasing peak systolic wall stress (Fig. 15), whereby coronary vascular reserves are normal when systolic wall stress is normal or reduced, comparable to those in hypertrophic obstructive cardiomyopathy [49, 50,

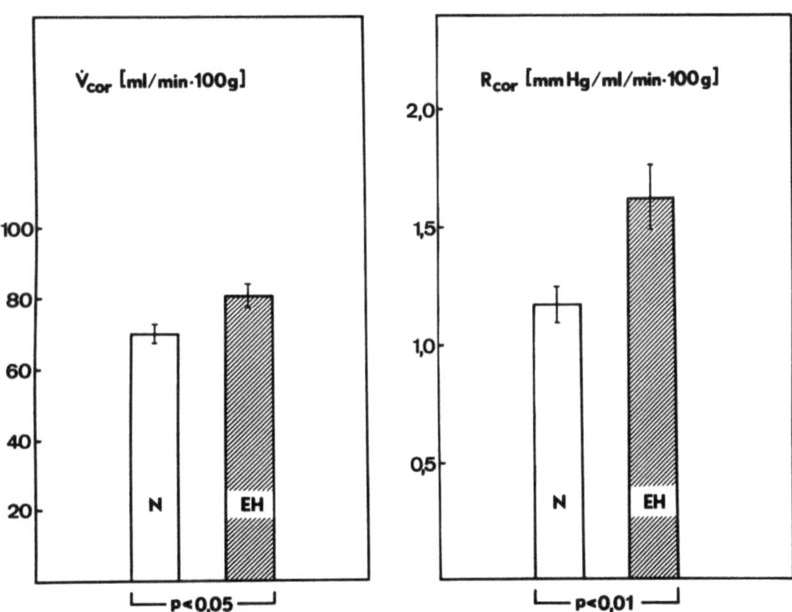

Fig. 12. Coronary blood flow ($\dot{V}_{cor}$) and coronary vascular resistance (R_{cor}) in essential hypertension

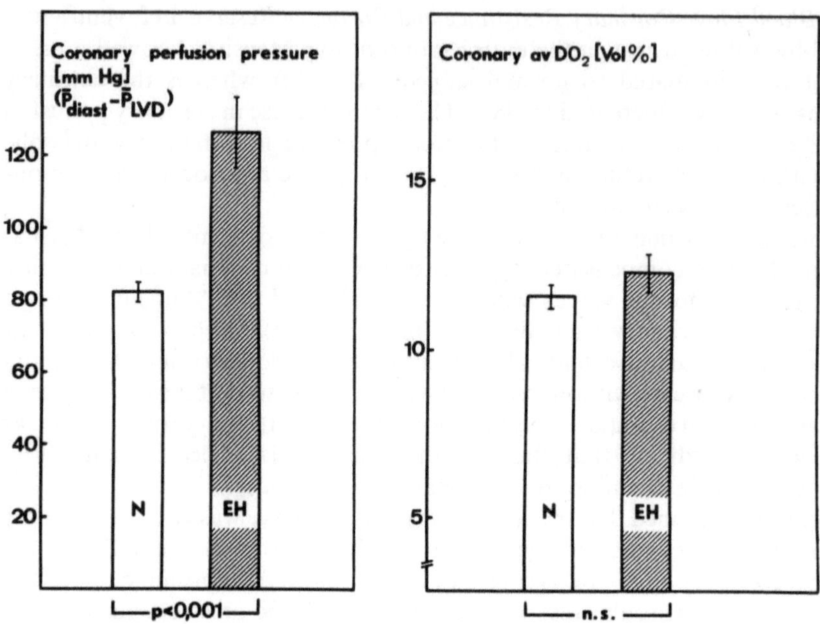

Fig. 13. Coronary perfusion pressure and arteriocoronary venous oxygen difference in essential hypertension

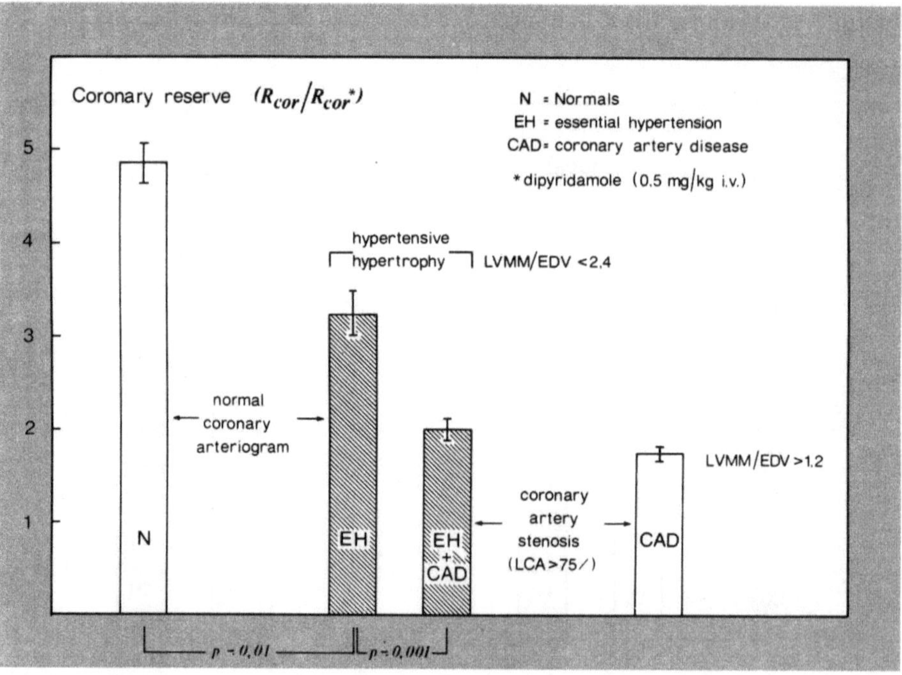

Fig. 14. Coronary reserve in normal subjects, in essential hypertension without coronary stenoses, in essential hypertension with coronary stenoses and in normotensive coronary artery disease. Note the considerable decrease even in those essential hypertensives with normal coronary arteriograms

Table 5. Coronary perfusion pressure (P_{cor}), arteriocoronary venous oxygen difference (avDO$_2$), left ventricular coronary blood flow ($\dot{V}_{cor}$) and coronary vascular resistance (R_{cor}) in 12 normal subjects, 63 patients with essential hypertension (EH) and 38 patients with coronary artery disease (CAD)

		P_{cor} [mm Hg]	avDO$_2$ [Vol%]	$\dot{V}_{cor}$ [ml/min · 100 g]	R_{cor} [mm Hg · min · 100 g · ml^{-1}]
Normals	(n = 12)	82 ± 2	12.2 ± 0.1	71 ± 3	1.15 ± 0.04
EH	(n = 63)	129 ± 8***	12.9 ± 0.2	83 ± 2**	1.57 ± 0.06***
CHD	(n = 38)	87 ± 5	12.8 ± 0.6	64 ± 3*	1.36 ± 0.09

* p < 0.02 ** p < 0.005 *** p < 0.001

94], and are reduced when systolic wall stress is increased. For high systolic wall stress the mass-volume ratio was generally lower than for low systolic wall stress. However, no tendency in any direction could be detected in the relationship between the left ventricular coronary vascular reserve and the degree of hypertrophy, which can be assessed on the basis of the mass-volume ratio.

Oxygen Consumption of the Left Ventricle. The oxygen consumption of the whole left ventricle (ml/min) in the entire group of hypertensives increased by 62% compared to normal subjects (Fig. 16 a). There was a linear relationship to the left ventricular

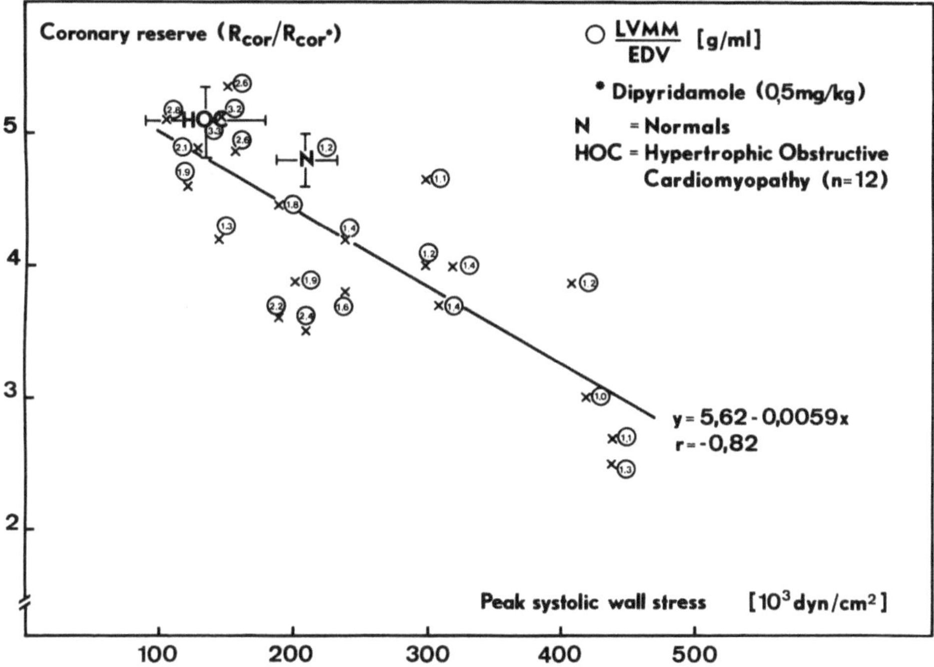

Fig. 15. Relationship between the peak systolic wall stress and the coronary reserve of the left ventricle. Note how the coronary reserve decreases with increasing systolic wall stress

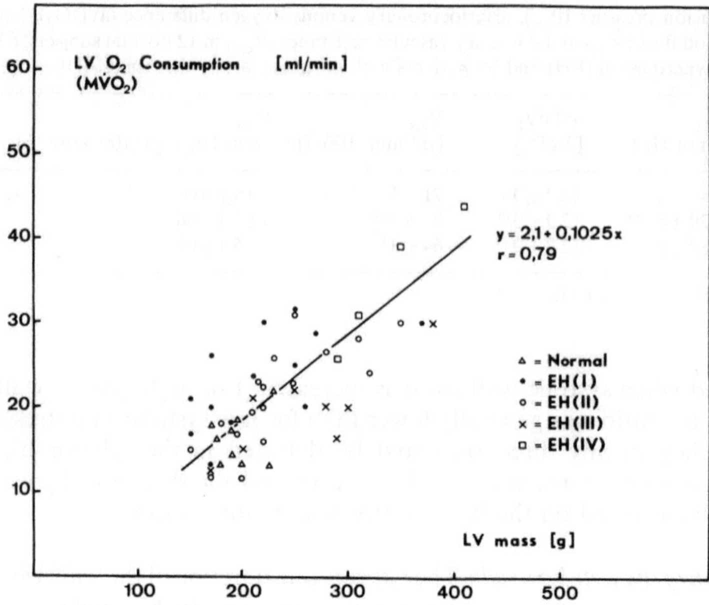

Fig. 16a. Relationship between the absolute left ventricular muscle mass and the oxygen consumption of the whole left ventricle. Note that there is a satisfactory relationship between the two variables

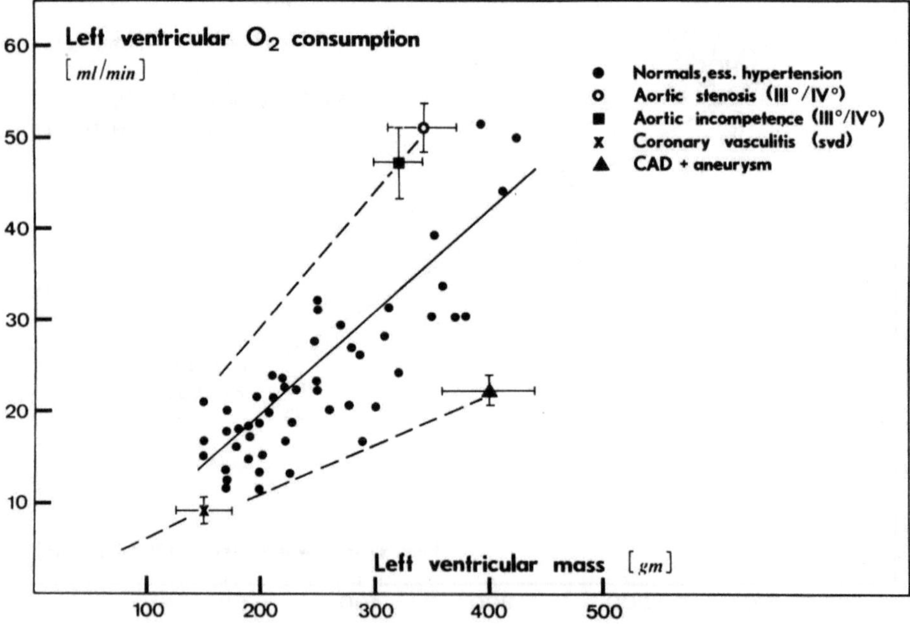

Fig. 16b. Relationship between left ventricular mass and left ventricular oxygen consumption. svd, small vessel disease

28

muscle mass (r = 0.79; Fig. 16 a), so that the increasing oxygen consumption in essential hypertension is a function of ventricular hypertrophy and the underlying pressure load.

When considering other types of left ventricular overload (aortic stenosis, aortic incompetence) or diseases with altered coronary function (coronary artery disease, small vessel disease on the basis of coronary vasculitis), the total left ventricular oxygen consumption also seemed to be linearly correlated with the total left ventricular muscle mass (Fig. 16 b).

There was poor correlation between $M\dot{V}O_2$ and ventricular function (as manifested by cardiac index, stroke work index, external cardiac work, pressure-time index, isovolumic contractility indices, ejection phase indices, systolic pressure and other measures).

The mass-volume ratio was inversely related to $M\dot{V}O_2$ (Fig. 17). At isobaric conditions, the largest mass-volume ratio and lowest $M\dot{V}O_2$ was found in patients with hypertrophic obstructive cardiomyopathy, while in those with decompensated aortic stenosis and aortic incompetence the lowest mass-volume ratio was associated with the largest $M\dot{V}O_2$. Normotensive patients with normal left ventricular function or with coronary artery disease had a lower $M\dot{V}O_2$ at a comparable mass-volume ratio.

Because the mass-volume ratio, at equal systolic pressure, represents the major determinant of peak systolic wall stress, correlation was performed between peak systolic wall stress and the $M\dot{V}O_2$. A significant relationship was found between

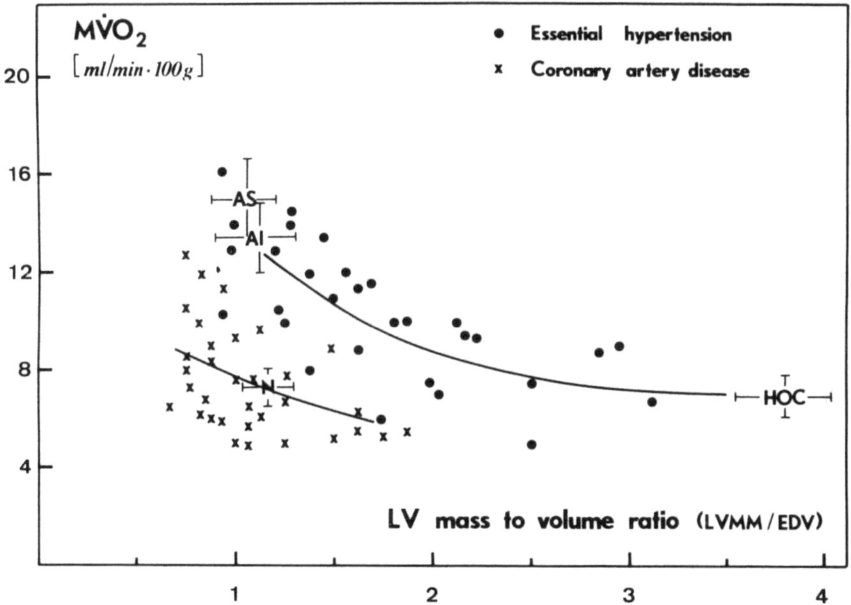

Fig. 17. Relationship between left ventricular (LV) mass-volume ratio (LVMM/EDV) and left ventricular oxygen consumption per weight unit ($M\dot{V}O_2$). *AI* aortic incompetence; *AS* aortic stenosis; *HOC* hypertrophic obstructive cardiomyopathy

them (Figs. 18–21) Patients with decompensated aortic stenosis and aortic incompetence were within the upper range, and the normotensive normal subjects were within the lower range of this relationship. Extrapolation to zero stress resulted in an intercept of 3.28 ml/min × 100 g (Fig. 20). This value, although somewhat increased, corresponds quite well with the oxygen consumption of the empty beating heart. Steepness of this regression indicates an increase in $M\dot{V}O_2$ by 2.8 ml/min × 100 g for an increase in peak systolic wall stress by $100 \, (10^3 \, \mathrm{dyn/cm^2})$ for normal subjects as well as for those with coronary artery disease and hypertrophic heart disease. As can further be seen from this correlation, oxygen consumption can, however, also be reduced or normal in essential hypertension as compared with normotensive left ventricles. In these cases there may be either an inadequate hypertrophy with increased mass-volume ratio and reduced peak systolic wall stress or an adequate hypertrophy which can keep the peak systolic wall stress at normal values with high systolic pressure due to a proportional increase in the mass-volume ratio. The mean myocardial oxygen consumption is thus increased in essential hypertension and is largely determined by the individual degree of hypertrophy, i. e. by the relationship between muscle mass, volume and wall stress.

The lowest peak systolic wall stress, which was found in patients with chronic hypertensive hypertrophy, was $100 \pm 12 \, (10^3 \, \mathrm{dyn/cm^2})$ and the largest peak systolic

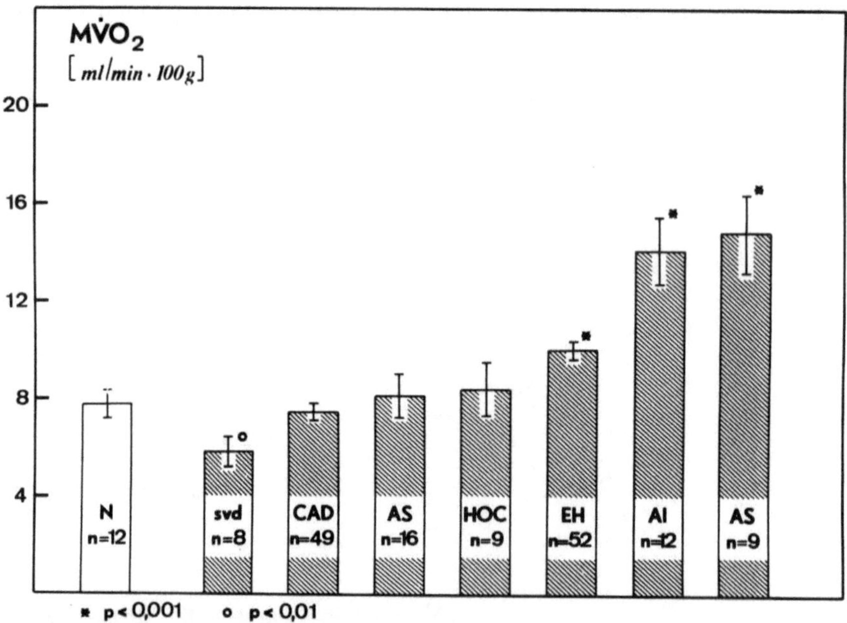

Fig. 18. Myocardial oxygen consumption per left ventricular weight unit in hypertensive hypertrophy and in non-hypertensive left ventricular hypertrophy. N, normals (normotensive, non-hypertrophied); SVD, small vessel disease, on the basis of coronary and systemic immune complex vasculitis; CAD, coronary artery disease; AS, aortic stenosis (NYHA I/II); HOC, hypertrophic obstructive cardiomyopathy; EH, essential hypertension; AI, aortic incompetence (NYHA III/IV); AS (*extreme right bar*), aortic stenosis (NYHA III/IV)

30

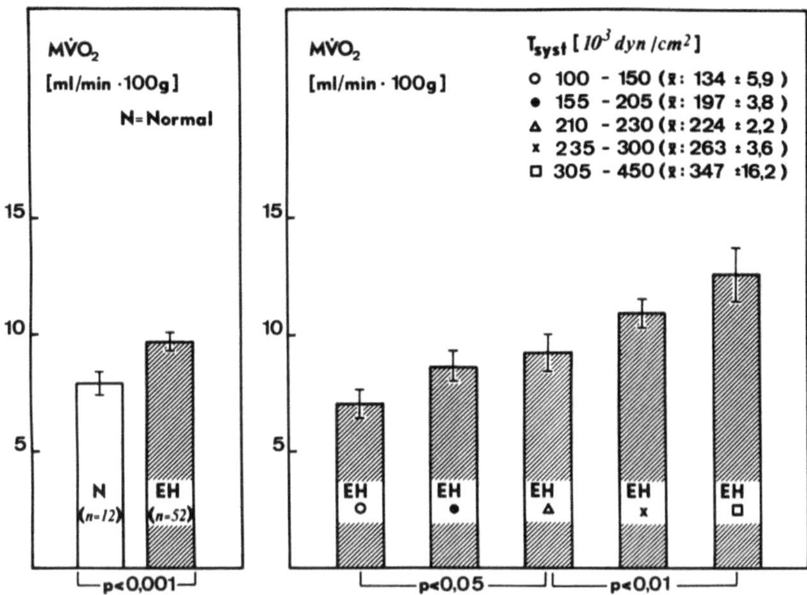

Fig. 19. Oxygen consumption of the left ventricle per unit of weight in essential hypertension. Note the significantly increased mean oxygen consumption in the entire group of hypertensives (*left*). Further note that graded changes in left ventricular oxygen consumption result if the peak systolic wall stress is taken into account

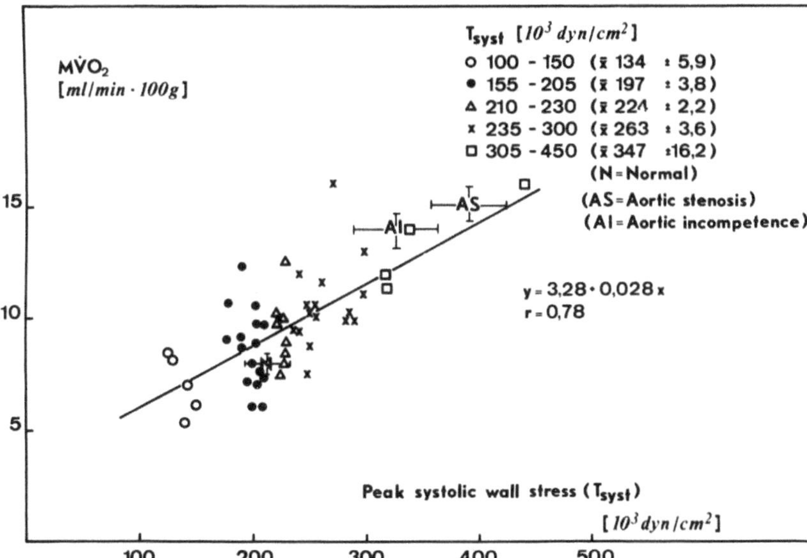

Fig. 20. Relationship between peak systolic wall stress and left ventricular oxygen consumption per weight unit (MV̇O₂). Note the significant relationship between both varaibles

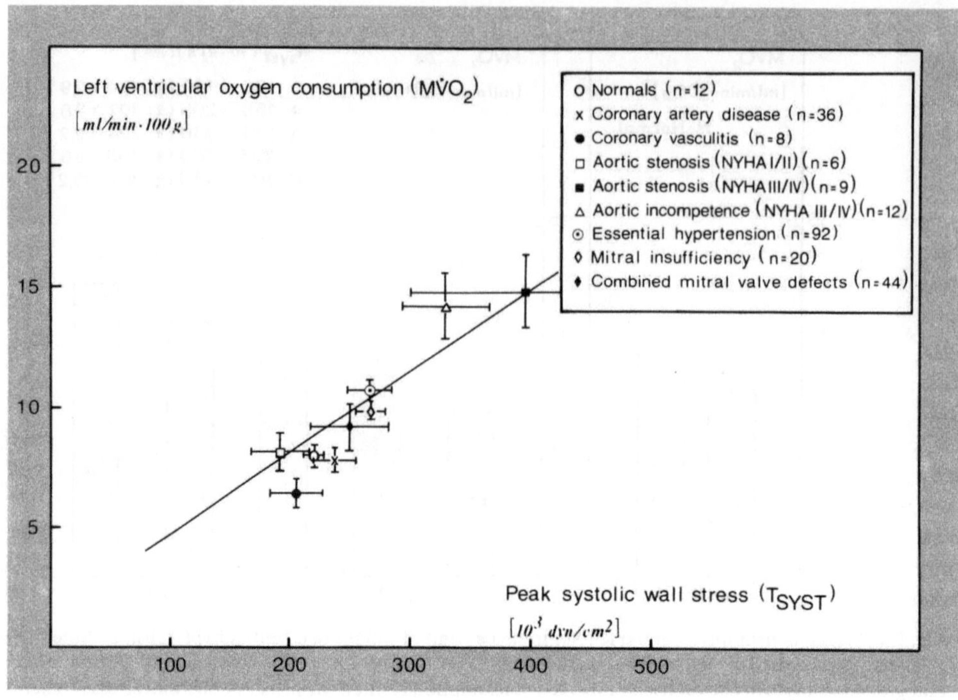

Fig. 21. Relationship between peak systolic wall stress (*abscissa*) and myocardial oxygen consumption (*ordinate*). Note that systolic wall stress, expressed per cross-sectional area, is linearly correlated with left ventricular oxygen consumption, expressed per left ventricular weight unit

wall stress was 450 ± 46 (Table 6). In comparison with the normal subjects (peak systolic wall stress $= 220 \pm 9 \times 10^3$ dyn/cm^2), patients with chronic hypertrophy may have a decreased, normal or increased peak systolic wall stress. Thus, both low and high stress hypertrophy may occur, the ratio between maximal and minimal stress averaging 4.5 (Table 6, Fig. 22).

Table 6. Minimal and maximal values of peak systolic wall stress

	Minimum	Maximum	$\dfrac{\text{Maximum}}{\text{Minimum}}$
T_{syst} (10^3 dyn/cm^2)[a]	100 $\pm$12	450$\pm$46	4.5 = stress reserve
$\dot{M}VO_2$ (ml/min $\times$ 100 g)[b]	5.2$\pm$ 0.3	24$\pm$ 2.9	4.6 = metabolic reserve
$\dot{V}_{cor}$ (ml/min $\times$ 100 g)[c]	79 $\pm$12	392$\pm$26	4.9 = coronary reserve

All values (maximal versus minimal) p < 0.001.

[a] Essential hypertension.

[b] Chronic valvular and hypertensive pressure overload.

[c] Normal subjects (before and after administration of dipyridamole, 0.5 mg/kg).

$\dot{M}VO_2$, myocardial oxygen consumption; T_{syst}, peak circumferential systolic wall stress; $\dot{V}_{cor}$, coronary blood flow.

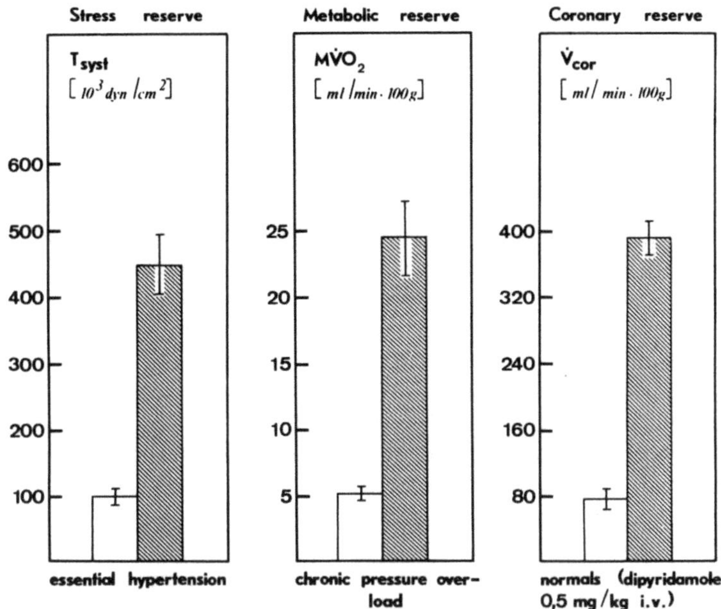

Fig. 22. Stress reserve (left), metabolic reserve (mid) and coronary reserve (right) in essential hypertension, in chronic pressure overload and in normals. Note the similarity in the 3 reserves determined

Discussion of the Results

Systolic wall stress is the consequence of changes in mass, ventricular volume and systolic pressure. In *acute* pressure overload, systolic stress increases in parallel with an increase in pressure because the mass-volume ratio (or wall thickness-radius ratio) remains nearly unaltered. In *chronic* pressure and volume overload, systolic stress is altered in accordance with chronically altered left ventricular geometry (mass-volume ratio). In either condition, systolic stress reflects the response in ventricular hypertrophy to the acute or chronic left ventricular overload. Therefore, left ventricular hypertrophy may be appropriate or inappropriate with regard to the systolic stress changes that depend on the mass or volume changes relative to load. This concept implies that systolic stress represents the afterload imposed on the left ventricular wall.

The increase in coronary blood flow per unit of weight (per 100 g of left ventricular weight) which was found in all essential hypertensives shows that with largely normal coronary oxygen extraction, as measured by the largely normal arteriocoronary venous oxygen difference, the myocardial blood flow must increase in order to be able to maintain an adequate oxygen balance in the left ventricle per unit of weight. Essential hypertension thus represents a cardiac disease and a type of hypertrophy which, in contrast to previously known types of cardiac hypertrophy [49–51, 58, 61, 93, 99, 107–109], such as those elicited by left ventricular pressure and volume loads (aortic and mitral valve lesions, congenital heart anomalies, A V shunt etc.), achieves a higher degree of moycardial or coronary blood flow and a

33

higher degree of myocardial oxygen consumption despite a significant increase in coronary vascular resistance. Generally, changes in the myocardial energy demand of the human heart are initiated by changes in coronary blood flow, since the arteriocoronary venous oxygen extraction is complete, i.e. maximal or sub-maximal [8, 58], and can only marginally be raised by further oxygen extraction. Consequently, under the conditions of an increase in myocardial oxygen consumption there is a reduction in coronary vascular resistance and a rise in coronary blood flow which meets the raised myocardial energy demand of the left ventricle. Diseases of the human heart accompanied by an increase in coronary blood flow and myocardial oxygen consumption and a simultaneous rise in coronary vascular resistance as seen in essential hypertension have not yet been reported. Thus it must be assumed that the left ventricle or the coronary vascular system in essential hypertension achieves or controls the increase in coronary blood flow required to meet the metabolic demands or the raised myocardial oxygen consumption against an abnormally increased coronary vascular resistance. Numerous considerations and findings have been reported on the possible causes of increased vascular resistance in essential hypertension [68]. It is conceivable that following a metabolic relief of the left ventricle, e. g. by antihypertensive measures or measures of negative inotropic effect, a further increase in coronary vascular resitance is to be expected [68], since under these conditions the decrease in coronary vascular resistance induced by metabolic factors is inhibited.

Quantitatively the impairment of the left ventricular coronary vascular reserve in essential hypertension with significant coronary stenoses ($> 75\%$) as determined by coronary angiography is comparable to that in normotensive coronary artery disease with a corresponding degree of stenosis [93]. In this respect, essential hypertension with coronary artery disease represents a syndrome of coronary findings which is similar to the impairment of the coronary vascular reserve and the coronary risk in normotensive coronary artery disease. In essential hypertension with coronary stenoses this results in a presumably even higher risk of ischaemia of the left ventricle than in normotensive coronary artery disease, since the decisive triggering condition for the development of angina pectoris and coronary insufficiency, i.e. disproportion between oxygen supply and demand, is considerably enhanced by the underlying systolic left ventricular pressure load. Thus there is a high risk of ischaemia in essential hypertension with coronary artery disease.

Even in compensated essential hypertension without coronary stenoses detectable by coronary angiography there is a marked impairment of the coronary vascular reserve of the left ventricle. Since in normal coronary angiograms this cannot be explained by the *coronary factor* as determined by gross examination, i. e. by coronary angiography, and since the *myocardial factor* as determined by estimating the degree of left ventricular hypertrophy, the mass-volume ratio of the left ventricle, the mass-volume ratio and the end-diastolic and peak systolic wall stresses do not correlate with the impairment of the coronary vascular reserve in essential hypertension without abnormal findings on coronary angiography, the conclusion is obvious that this functional disturbance in coronary regulation may be the result of an increase in the coronary vascular reserve due to an affection of the small intramural coronary arteries [43, 46]. It is not necessary to assume that there is a functional coronary constriction since histological examinations of the coronary vascular system in arterial hypertension have shown that the small arteries and arterioles exhibited thickened vascular wall structures, fibroses, scleroses and narrowed lumina [46]. The left ventricle in essential hypertension with normal coronary angiograms must thus be regarded as being at risk as regards the development of ischaemia, alone from the standpoint of the coronary regulatory capacity.

The impairment of the coronary reserve in these patients correlates with the clinical experience that patients with essential hypertension or patients with angina pectoris and essential hypertension may, even with normal coronary angiograms, have clinical complaints and objective symptoms similar to those in coronary artery disease. This means that the basic process of angina pectoris in essential hypertension with normal coronary angiograms may be a *functional* coronary micro-angiopathy [43, 46]. It must further be assumed that consistently raised blood pressure levels or intermittent peak levels result in an increase in the myocardial oxygen consumption which may lead to a critical situation in myocardial oxygen supply. Both factors, i.e. the impairment of the coronary regulatory capacity and the increase in the myocardial oxygen demand, may contribute to the pathogenesis of angina pectoris-like symptoms in essential hypertension with normal coronary angiograms.

The increase in oxygen consumption of the whole left ventricle in essential hypertension can be explained by the increase in the absolute left ventricular muscle mass. However, the increase in the relation between these two variables (left ventricular muscle mass, total oxygen consumption) varied considerably in the hypertension groups examined so that there were differences in the oxygen consumption per 100 g left ventricular weight. This means that apart from the mass-related increase in myocardial oxygen consumption there is also evidence of a mass-independent rise in the myocardial energy demand. This may be caused by an increase in the energy-determinating parameters of cardiac mechanics or ventricular function, of which the peak systolic wall stress is of paramount importance [99]. No correlation was found between the raised oxygen consumption per 100 g and the left ventricular pressure, pumping and inotropic parameters. Since wall stress depends on the intraventricular pressure, the thickness of the ventricular wall and the radius, the degree of hypertrophy or dilatation of the left ventricle together with the absolute change in mass following essential hypertension represents an important determinant of myocardial energy demand. With comparatively increasing arterial pressure a progressive ventricular dilatation is associated with a pathological decrease in the mass-volume ratio and an increase in the peak systolic wall stress. Subsequently the oxygen consumption rises. Thus even in normal coronary angiograms the triggering conditions are present for myocardial ischaemia or angina pectoris-like symptoms since a critical change in the degree of hypertrophy (myocardial factor) leads to a disproportion between oxygen supply and demand in essential hypertension. With a comparatively increasing arterial pressure load there thus exists a pathogenetic correlation between the end-diastolic volume or the size of the left ventricle and the change in the myocardial energy demand following the stress-induced hypertrophy or dilatation in essential hypertension. Clinically the ischaemic risk of the left ventricle must therefore be expected to increase with increasing ventricular dilatation.

The existence of both low and high stress hypertrophy in chronic heart disease may help to explain the difference in oxygen demands as well as the variable results that have been reported for left ventricular oxygen consumption in patients with a chronically hypertrophied heart. For example, in aortic stenosis a 4.14-fold variation in $M\dot{V}O_2$ has been reported (from 5.8 to 24 ml/min $\times$ 100 g). In essential hypertension the range of $M\dot{V}O_2$ extends from approximately 5.2 to 16 ml/min $\times$ 100 g (3.1-fold). These variations seem controversial and may be due in part to variations in heart rate, cardiac work or contractility. There is little question that contractility or acute inotropic interventions, or both, may modify the $M\dot{V}O_2$, although the role of contractility in influencing the overall oxygen consumption in the chronically diseased hypertrophic and failing human heart has not yet been clearly identified. It appears somewhat surprising that a large $M\dot{V}O_2$ was found in patients with the lowest values for left ventricular function and contractility and the lowest $M\dot{V}O_2$ was present in patients with normal left ventricular function and contractility, particularly in those with essential hypertension, who had significant increases in the maximal rate of pressure development (dP/dt_{max}). This result may be the consequence of a minor influence of contractility on overall $M\dot{V}O_2$ in chronic heart disease, or the result of a disproportionate interplay between the contractile state and systolic wall stress in favor of a dominant influence of peak systolic wall stress on cardiac oxygen demand. In a quantitative sense, systolic wall stress, as demonstrated by our study, may play the major role and may predominantly influence $M\dot{V}O_2$. Thus, a depressed contractile state may be associated with an increase in $M\dot{V}O_2$ when peak systolic wall stress is increased (essential hypertension group IV, aortic stenosis and aortic incompetence in functional classes III and IV), and decreased $M\dot{V}O_2$ may be present during normal contractility when peak systolic wall stress is decreased (essential hypertension group I, aortic stenosis and aortic incompetence in functional classes I and II).

Essential hypertension with progressive cardiac enlargement, as measured by the changes in heart size obtained from chest X-ray examinations, must therefore always be regarded as a hypertensive heart disease which involves a risk of ischaemia. This does not exclude the possibility that a left ventricle of normal or only moderately increased size in essential hypertension due to concurrently occurring coronary artery stenoses may not also involve an increased risk of ischaemia or myocardial infarction.

The metabolic reserve of the hypertrophic left ventricle following essential hypertension is already impaired under resting conditions with the myocardial consumption per unit of weight being increased. It is assumed that with increasing end-diastolic volume or with a decreasing mass-volume ratio, i. e. with progressive left ventricular enlargement, the metabolic reserve is increasingly impaired via an increase in the myocardial oxygen consumption. Therapeutic measures by which an effective reduction in blood pressure and heart size as well as an increase in the mass-volume ratio can be achieved may also improve the ventricular function, reduce the myocardial oxygen demand and increase the mechanical and metabolic reserves of the left ventricle. Thus the *heart size* in essential hypertension not only represents a criterion of the ventricular function but also a useful correlative of the level of the myocardial energy demand and the ischaemic risk of the left ventricle.

36

3.3 Regional Degree of Hypertrophy and Proportionality
   of Ventricular Wall Hypertrophy

It is the purpose of this chapter to analyse the regional left ventricular hypertrophy
in a larger sample of patients with essential hypertension by taking into account
measurements of the regional wall thickness, the shortening of the hemiaxes,
regional wall stresses and changes in the thickness of the ventricular wall.

The trials were performed in 92 patients with essential hypertension. All results
obtained from the hypertension groups were compared with those from a group of
normal patients (n = 12) in whom the presence of heart anomalies was excluded by
cardiac catheterisation and who did not show hypertrophy, hypertension, vitia or
coronary artery stenoses.

Results

Case Material. In 13 (14%) of the 92 patients examined an irregularly hypertrophied
anterior wall of the left ventricle was found, i. e. they had an asymmetric ventricular
configuration predominantly in the middle of the ventricle or at the site of the
ventricular function located towards the apex (Table 7). Quantitative ventriculography in these 13 patients showed a largely normal end-diastolic volume (EDV

Table 7. Case material. Historical data and clinical symptoms of the 13 hypertensives with irregular
ventricular wall hypertrophy. Note the high percentage with angina pectoris and its response to
propranolol

Irregular ventricular wall hypertrophy in essential hypertension	
Number	n = 13 (out of 92) (14%)
Age (years)	39
Severity [122]	II
Optic fundus [47]	II
Duration of hypertension (years)	> 6
Exertional cardiac insufficiency	n = 5 (38%)
Cardiac insufficiency at rest	−
Angina pectoris	n = 13 (100%)
Cardiac dysrhythmias	n = 1 (VES)
Left ventricular hypertrophy (chest X-ray)	n = 8 (62%)
(ECG)	n = 13 (100%)
Left atrial hypertrophy (ECG)	n = 10 (77%)
Coronary stenoses (°III, LCA)	n = 9 (69%)
Non-cardiac vascular stenoses	n = 2 (15%)
Systolic heart murmurs	n = 8 (62%)
Delayed systoles	n = 5 (38%)
Special cardiac sounds	n = 2 (15%)
Challenge tests (amyl nitrite etc.)	−
Ventriculo-arterial pressure gradient	−
Response to propranolol: angina pectoris	n = 13 (100%)
Hypertension	n = 10 (77%)

$= 92 \pm 3$ ml/m^2) with the end-systolic volume being normal or reduced (ESV $= 21$ ± 1 ml/m^2) (Table 8). Qualitatively the ventriculograms were characterised by an asymmetric shape in the end-diastole with in part completely irregular ventricular configurations (Fig. 23).

Formally there were striking similarities to be found to the ventriculograms obtained from patients with hypertrophic obstructive cardiomyopathy. However, neither measurements of the intraventricular pressure nor challenge tests (Valsalva test, amyl nitrite inhalation, post-extrasystolic potentiation) indicated in any case the presence of an obstruction of haemodynamic effect, i.e. a ventriculo-arterial pressure gradient. Right coronary angiograms which were obtained from each patient showed a normal right ventricular contraction function. Nine of these patients had severe angina pectoris with coronary stenoses as verified by coronary angiography (grades II–IV) [54]. Two patients also had carotic artery stenoses requiring surgery. It was known that arterial hypertension had been present in all patients for more than 6 years. It should be mentioned that in these patients angina pectoris and hypertension responded remarkably to propranolol (Table 7).

Regional Degree of Hypertrophy. In order to quantify the degree, extent and regularity of regional hypertrophy, the regional wall thickness values and the end-diastolic/end-systolic wall thickness changes were analysed in the five ventricular segments (Fig. 24). In all patients examined the end-diastolic as well as the end-systolic thickness of the anterior wall of the left ventricle was greatest at the base of the heart. The thickness decreased up to the ventricular equator, where it reached its minimum, and thereafter increased towards the apex. The differences in regional wall thickness at the end-diastole or end-systole were smallest in decompensated hypertensives with left ventricular dilatation and were greatest in compensated hypertensives with concentric hypertrophy and coronary stenoses as determined by coronary angiography (Figs. 25 and 26).

Table 8. Ventricular dynamics and geometry in 12 normal patients and in the 13 patients with irregular ventricular wall hypertrophy. EH, essential hypertension; IRVH, irregular ventricular wall hypertrophy; EDV, end-diastolic volume; ESV, end-systolic volume; SV, stroke volume; EF, ejection fraction; d_{diast}, diastolic wall thickness; $\triangle$-wall thickness, percentage change of the ventricular wall thickness related to the end-diastolic intitial value ($=100\%$); T_{syst}, peak circumferential systolic wall stress of the left ventricle; T_{diast}, end-diastolic circumferential wall stress of the left ventricle

	Normals (n = 12)	EH ± IRVH (n = 13)
EDV (ml/m^2)	82 ±4	92 ± 3
ESV (ml/m^2)	24 ±2	21 ± 1
SV (ml/m^2)	64 ±3	71 ± 3
EF (%)	73 ±	77
d_{diast} (cm/m^2)	0.62 ± 0.02	0.91 ± 0.06
d_{syst} (cm/m^2)	0.98 ± 0.05	2.12 ± 0.09
$\triangle$-wall thickness	+ 58	+ 133
T_{syst} (10^3 dyn/cm^2)	221 ±27	142 ±39
T_{diast} (10^3 dyn/cm^2)	27 ± 8	30 ± 3

The maximal thickening of the anterior wall of the left ventricle during the course of a cardiac action, i.e. the end-diastolic/end-systolic change in wall thickness, was greatest in the region of the apically directed equator (M, M_3) (Figs. 25 and 26). This means that the ventricular wall region with the greatest end-diastolic/end-systolic change in distance and the greatest hemiaxis shortening also showed the greatest relative increase in ventricular wall thickness during a cardiac cycle. The increase in wall thickness measured in this ventricular wall region was, within the hypertension groups, greatest in compensated hypertensives with coronary artery disease proven by coronary angiography (Fig. 26). Hence this group revealed the greatest relative differences in the regional end-diastolic/end-systolic wall thickness changes and it is in these cases where the highest degree of asymmetry or irregularity of the ventricular wall hypertrophy, particularly in the middle of the ventricle, is to be expected.

The analysis of the regional wall stress showed that the end-diastolic and end-systolic wall stresses were highest at the equatorial circumference of the left ventricle, i.e. in that ventricular region with the greatest ventricular radius during diastole and systole and the smallest wall thickness during diastole (Figs. 27 and 28). Within the compensated hypertension groups the peak systolic wall stress in all five ventricular wall segments examined was considerably lower in those patients with irregular hypertrophy than in those with regular hypertrophy. Furthermore, the wall stress gradient from the base to the equator and from the equator to the apex was flattened and less marked than in regular hypertrophy. On the other hand, the decompensated hypertensives showed an even greater adjustment to the regional wall stress, so that with increasing ventricular dilatation a numerical adjustment of the wall thickness and wall stress and thus of the regional afterload of the left ventricle can be expected.

Discussion of the Results

The present studies have shown that in 14% of the essential hypertensives there was a significant irregular hypertrophy of the ventricular wall of ventriculogeometric effect. Since essential hypertension is one of the most common diseases, according to present knowledge it is also the most frequent cause of asymmetric or irregular ventricular hypertrophy or ventricular wall hypertrophy.

Although there was no uniformity in the location of the ventricular wall asymmetry in essential hypertension, wall segments located in the middle of the ventricle (M) or in the apical third of the ventricle (M_3) were predominantly involved. In none of the cases examined was an asymmetrie hypertrophy found in the basal third of the ventricle (M_1, M_2). The shape of the abnormally hypertrophy ventricular wall segment was irregular, i.e. unpredictable and non-uniform, with the anterior wall, and predominantly the middle of the ventricle (M) and the apical third (M_3), being involved in all cases. In four cases an hourglass-like circular wall thickening was found in the middle of the ventricle (M).

Hypertrophic obstructive cardiomyopathy is the prototype of an asymmetric or irregular ventricular wall hypertrophy [24, 35, 50, 94, 119]. In this disease the ventricular septum, the subaortic outflow tract or all other segments of the left

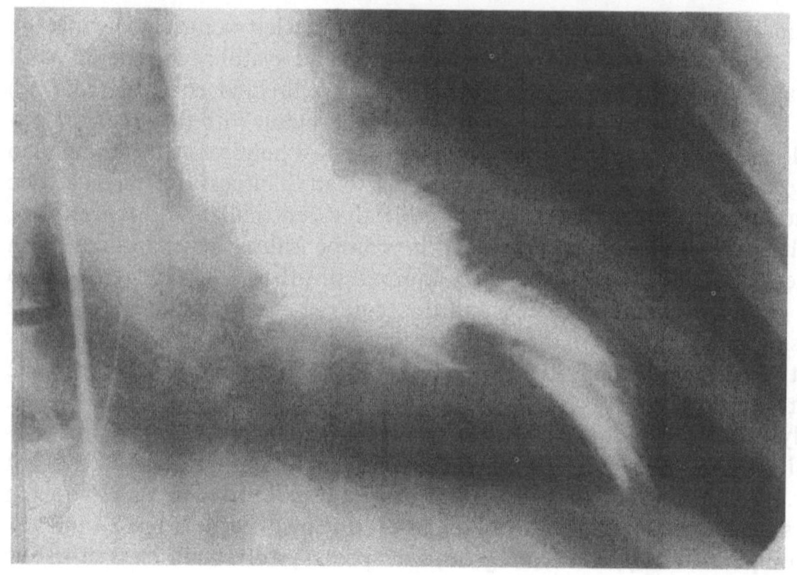

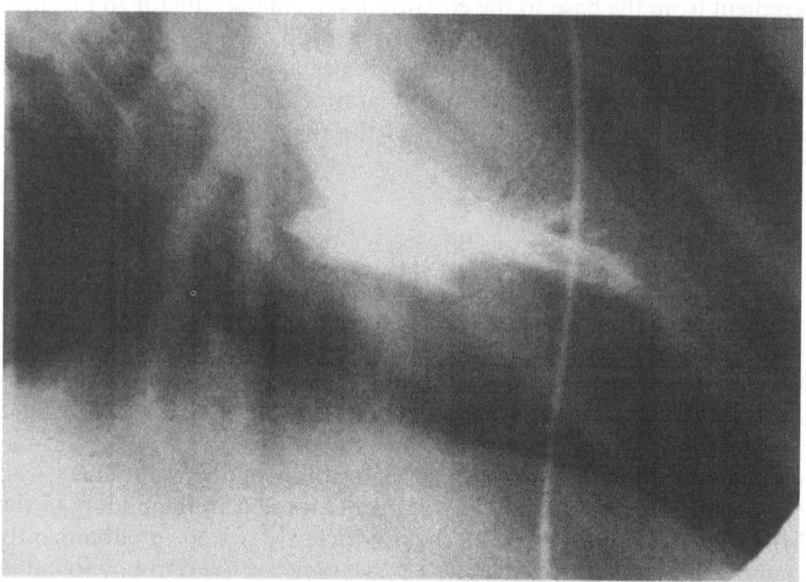

Fig. 23 a–d. Ventriculograms of two patients with irregular or asymmetric ventricular wall hypertrophy in essential hypertension

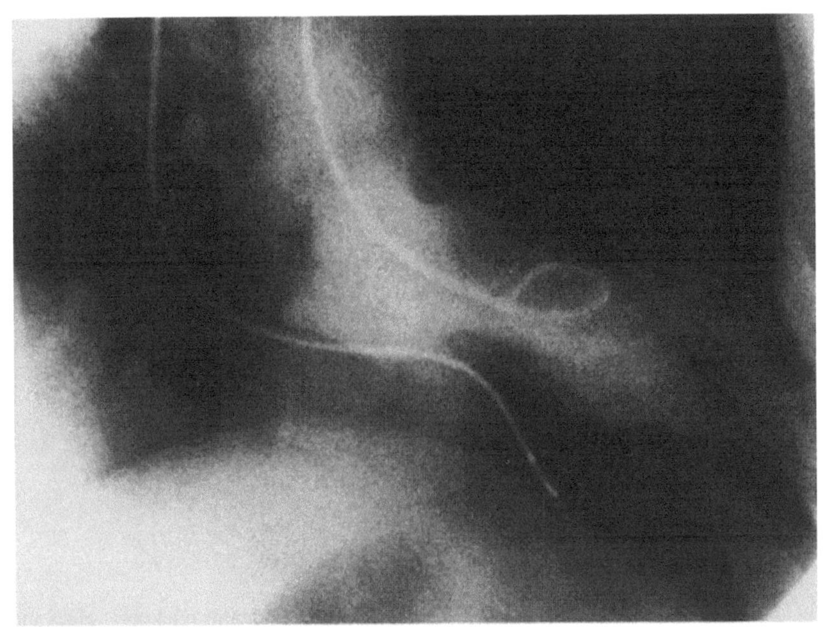

c

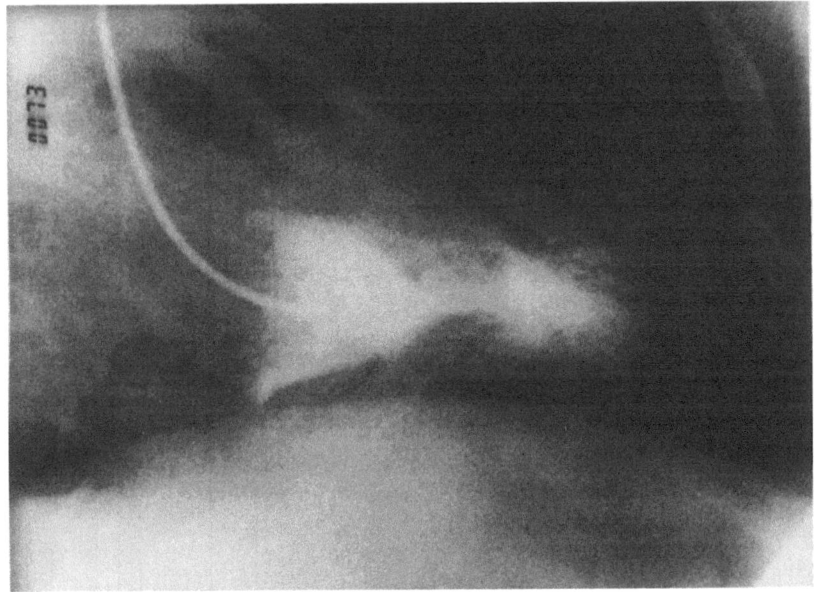

d

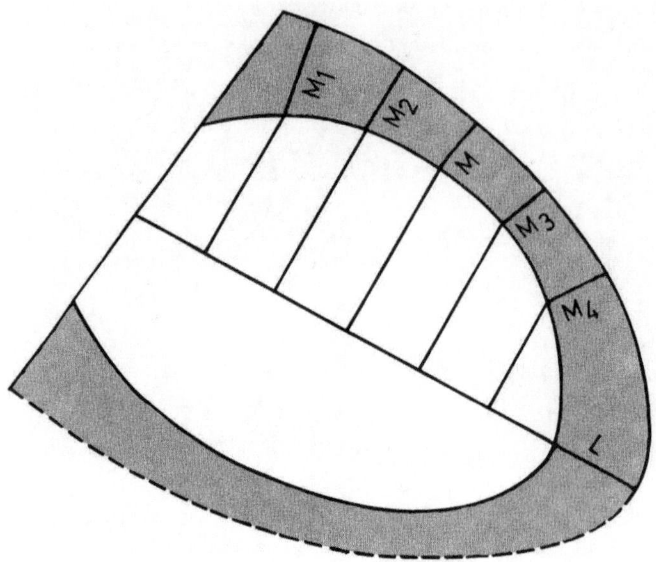

Fig. 24. Basic scheme for the evaluation of the hemiaxes and wall thickness values in five different ventricular wall segments

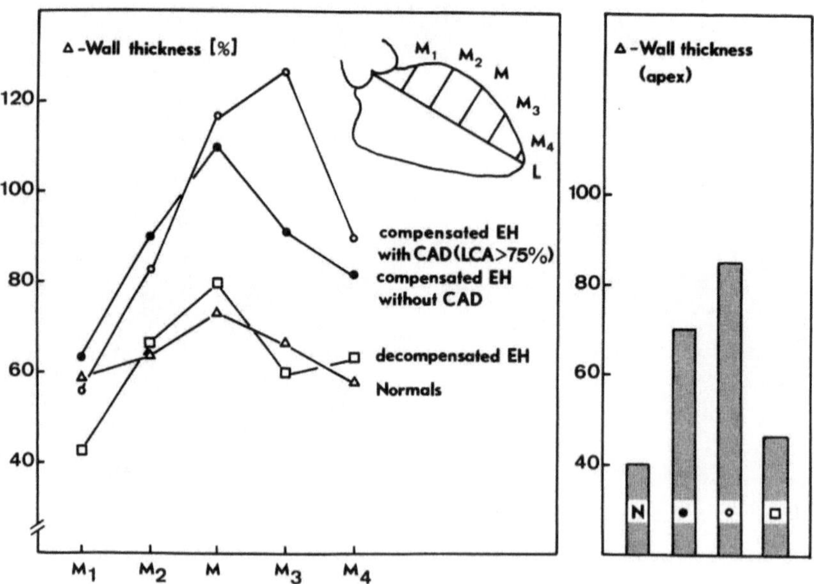

Fig. 25. Percentage wall thickness changes (end-diastolic/end-systolic) in the hypertension groups examined

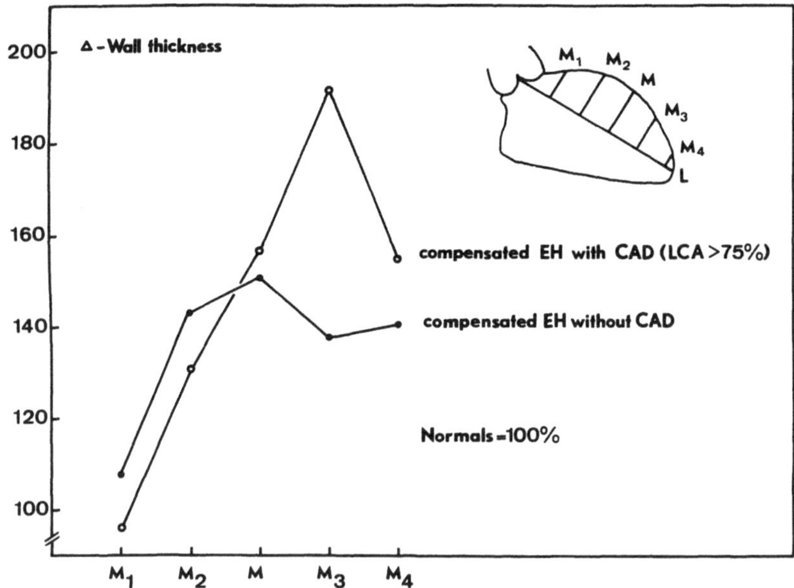

Fig. 26. Percentage wall thickness changes (end-diastolic/end-systolic) in compensated hypertensives with and without coronary artery disease. Normal value = 100%

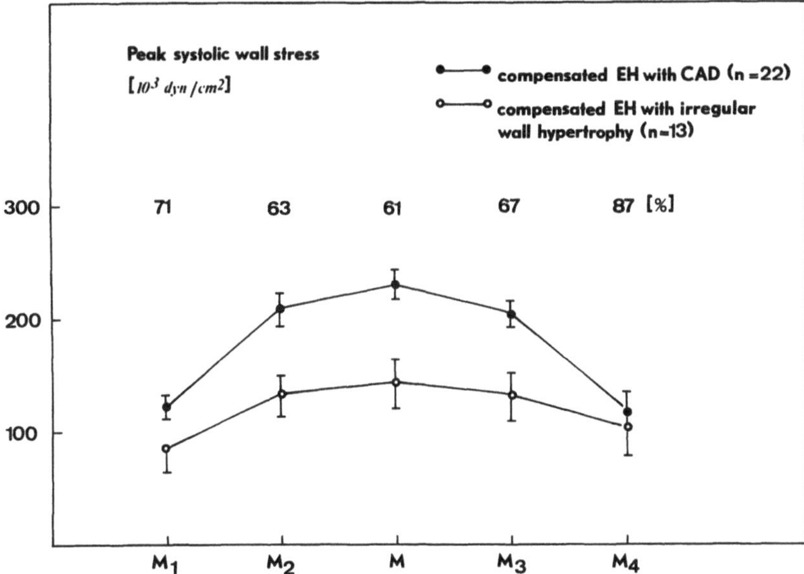

Fig. 27. Peak circumferential systolic wall stress in compensated essential hypertensives with coronary artery disease (n = 22) and in 13 patients with irregular ventricular wall hypertrophy. The figures show the percentages of the peak systolic wall stress in the 13 patients with irregular ventricular wall hypertrophy related to the wall stress values from the compensated hypertensives without irregular ventricular hypertrophy (= 100%)

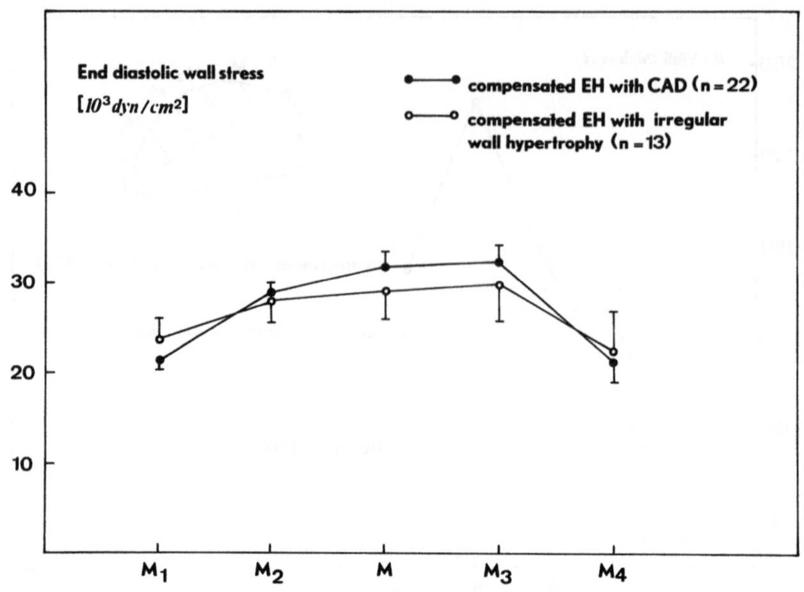

Fig. 28. Peak circumferential end-diastolic wall stress of the left ventricle in 22 compensated hypertensives with coronary artery disease and regular ventricular wall hypertrophy and in 13 patients with essential hypertension and irregular ventricular wall hypertrophy. Note the similar values for the end-diastolic wall stress in all ventricular wall segments

ventricle can be affected by the asymmetric hypertrophy. All intermediate stages are possible from light forms showing only a ghost of an 'hourglass' left ventricle without a ventriculo-arterial pressure gradient and negative challenge test results to most severe forms of intraventricular obstruction with high pressure gradients, positive challenge tests and angina pectoris. However, arterial hypertension in hypertrophic obstructive cardiomyopathy is found in only 1%–3% of cases. It is unlikely that there is a connection between the two diseases (essential hypertension and hypertrophic obstructive cardiomyopathy). Coronary stenoses are rare, and the coronary dynamics are largely normal [24, 50, 94, 119]. However, in none of the hypertensives examined was there an intraventricular obstruction, despite a considerable degree of irregularity of the ventricular hypertrophy. The challenge tests were negative. The right ventricle and the outflow tract of the right ventricle were normal. The coronary vascular reserve of the left ventricle was reduced to less than half the normal value. The majority of patients showed significant coronary stenoses of the left coronary artery. Thus it is not very likely from the clinical findings that the irregular ventricular wall hypertrophy in essential hypertension with respect to the presence or absence of an intraventricular obstruction merely represents an asymptomatic type of hypertrophic obstructive cardiomyopathy with essential hypertension. This would imply that the two diseases have aetiological factors in common, for which there is no evidence. It must rather be assumed that the irregular hypertrophy in essential hypertension shows a formal development which may result in ventriculograms similar to those obtained in hypertrophic

44

obstructive cardiomyopathy. From this it must not necessarily be deduced that a connection exists between the two conditions.

Analysis of the regional end-diastolic/end-systolic wall thickness changes of the left ventricle reveals that it is possible to record an irregular hypertrophy, i.e. irregular wall thickness changes, by measuring the regional thickness of the wall. It must be noted here that quantitatively excessive measurements are obtained for the wall thickness at M_1 (base of the heart) and M_4 as well as at L (apex) due to the filming and evaluation techniques chosen. However, this numerical overrating, which in the M_1, M_4 and L projections amounts to about 15%–25%, is largely constant, so that a group comparison between normal patients, hypertensives with regular hypertrophy and hypertensives with irregular hypertrophy is justified if the technique applied is kept constant.

The information available from literature on the regional wall thickness or the contraction patterns does not permit a final judgement on the extent of the end-diastolic/end-systolic wall thickness changes, i.e. on the increase in wall thickness during systole in normal subjects and in cardiac patients [16, 20–22, 36, 41, 57, 63, 77]: In animal experiments wall thickness changes of between 10% and 80% were reported; in normal patients the wall thickness increase measured at the equatorial circumference varies between 20% and 150%. In the normal patients examined in this study the mean end-diastolic/end-systolic wall thickness change at the equator was 58% and it decreased towards the base as well as towards the apex with increasing end-diastolic wall thickness. This means that the circumference with the greatest movement of the hemiaxis and the highest regional ejection fraction also showed the greatest regional wall thickness increase during systole. In contrast to the normal patients and the hypertensives with regular ventricular wall hypertrophy, the hypertensives with irregular hypertrophy showed excessive wall thickness increases by a maximal average of 133% (M) with a corresponding shortening of the hemiaxes in this area. In contrast, the wall thickness changes in the basal and apical ventricular segments were considerably smaller. Thus the wall thickness change at the base of the heart (M_1) in normal patients was 28%, in compensated hypertensives with regular ventricular wall hypertrophy, 37% and in compensated hypertensives with irregular ventricular wall hypertrophy, 41%. Corresponding relationships were found for the wall thickness changes at the apex. This means that the regional wall thickening at the base in normal patients and hypertensives with irregular hypertrophy only differed by a factor of 1.46, whereas at the equator the wall thickness change in hypertensives with irregular hypertrophy was 2.29 times that in normals.

The fact that the wall thickness change is greater at the equator than it is at both the base and the apex of the heart shows that the peak systolic wall stress measured at the equator (M) with closely similar end-diastolic volumes and comparable systolic pressure loads was regionally (M) smaller in hypertensives with irregular hypertrophy than in normal patients and in hypertensives with regular hypertrophy. Thus the peak systolic wall stress at the equator (M) in hypertensives with irregular hypertrophy at 142 (10^3 dyn/cm^2) only reached 61% of the peak systolic wall stress in normals. Hence the peak systolic wall stress is, despite a high degree of systolic pressure load of the left ventricle, kept low in a hypercompensatory manner as a consequence of irregular hypertrophy. On the other hand, there is a relative increase in the circumferential peak systolic wall stress towards the base and apex of the heart so that the peak systolic wall stress at the base amounts to 71% and at the apex to 87% of that in normals. The differences in the wall stress profiles above all appear to be the result of the different types of ventricular wall hypertrophy, which result in a specific pattern of wall thickness, wall thickness changes, regional muscle mass and wall stress which is typical of the irregular hypertrophy in essential hypertension.

Possible causes of the irregular ventricular hypertrophy in essential hypertension are in particular the extent, degree and duration of the arterial left ventricular pressure load. Furthermore a possible association with coronary stenoses and regional perfusion disorders and subsequent myocardial ischaemia must be taken into account. For the left ventricle the arterial pressure load, i. e. the ventricular afterload, is greatest at the equator (M) since the circumferential wall stress of the ventricle achieved during systole at this circumference is the greatest of all. This circumference of the left ventricle is thus exposed to the greatest mechanical stress from the standpoint of ventricular mechanics and geometry and was exactly that region where the irregularity of left ventricular hypertrophy was greatest, i. e. where the greatest wall thickness changes were observed during the systole when comparing them to those in normals and in other hypertension groups. An over-proportional end-diastolic wall thickness increase, as present in 14% of all hypertensives examined, would be appropriate to keep the peak systolic wall stress at normal or physiologically low levels, even under conditions of extremely high peak pressure loads and of comparable ventricular dimensions. Without a compensatory ventricular wall hypertrophy the peak equatorial systolic wall stress would, e. g. in acute hypertensive crises with the blood pressure increasing to twice the initial level, show a comparable increase. This would, however, also be accompanied by approximate doubling of the myocardial oxygen consumption. An over-proportional increase in the left ventricular wall thickness at the equatorial circumference might help to keep the maximal systolic afterload and the myocardial energy demand at this critical ventriculogeometric region at normal or low levels, even if there are extreme pressure loads. Correspondingly, the irregular or asymmetric hypertrophy of the left ventricle may be considered to be a compensatory mechanism which even under high pressure loads might help to maintain normal wall stress, afterload and energy balance conditions.

3.4 Determinants of Left Ventricular Hypertrophy and Diastolic Compliance

The aim of these investigations was to obtain information on the determinants of the degree of left ventricular hypertrophy in essential hypertension and on the relationships between degree of hypertrophy and left ventricular compliance and between degree of hypertrophy, compliance and ventricular function.

Results

Case Material (Table 9). Of 74 patients included in this study, 59 (80%) suffered from manifest angina pectoris and 32 (44%) had significant stenoses of coronary arteries.

46

Table 9. Case material

Number of patients		74
Age (years)		41
Degree of severity [122]		I–III
Duration of hypertension (years)		>2
Angina pectoris		n = 59 (80%)
Dyspnoea on exertion		n = 33 (45%)
Dyspnoea at rest		n = 18 (24%)
Condition following myocardial infarction		n = 21 (28%)
Condition following cerebral haemorrhage		n = 2 (3%)
Left ventricular hypertrophy (chest X-ray)		n = 63 (85%)
	(ECG)	n = 69 (93%)
Left atrial hypertrophy	(ECG)	n = 52 (70%)
Systolic cardiac murmurs		n = 38 (51%)
Extracardial bruits		n = 11 (15%)
Coronary stenoses	LCA > 75%	n = 22 (30%)
	LCA, RCA > 75%	n = 10 (14%)

Case histories or ECG recording revealed older myocardial infarctions in 21 patients. Signs of left ventricular hypertrophy were seen in almost all cases (85%–93%), so that there was a good correlation between left ventricular hypertrophy determined by means of ECG or X-ray and hypertrophy of the left ventricle determined by means of ventriculography. In 49 patients (68%) cardiac murmurs and extracardial bruits were heard, the latter mainly over the carotid arteries and the abdomen. No case of renal artery stenosis occurred. Two patients had experienced ischaemic cerebral haemorrhage several years prior to this investigation.

End-diastolic Wall Stress and Ventricular Compliance. In patients with compensated hypertension with and without coronary stenoses and regional wall contraction disturbances the end-diastolic wall stress was within normal limits, whereas in patients with decompensated hypertension it increased considerably (Fig. 29). There was a significant dependence of end-diastolic wall stress on end-diastolic volume, a linear regression being assumed between the two variables for the sake of simplicity (Fig. 30).

The good relationship between the two parameters can be explained by the increase in the inner ventricular radius which sets in with increasing diastolic volume and the increase in end-diastolic pressure which is mostly present in such cases.

Most of complicance and stiffness indices revealed a concordant (dP/dV, LMFS) or inverse (dV/dP, dV/dP · V) relation to the end-diastolic wall stress (T_{diast}) (Table 10). From these indices it was not possible to obtain more information on left ventricular compliance than that included in the conclusions drawn from end-diastolic wall stress values. However, these indices allowed the various hypertension groups to be defined somewhat more precisely. Accordingly, compliance of the left ventricle can shown to be largely normal in patients with compensated hyper-

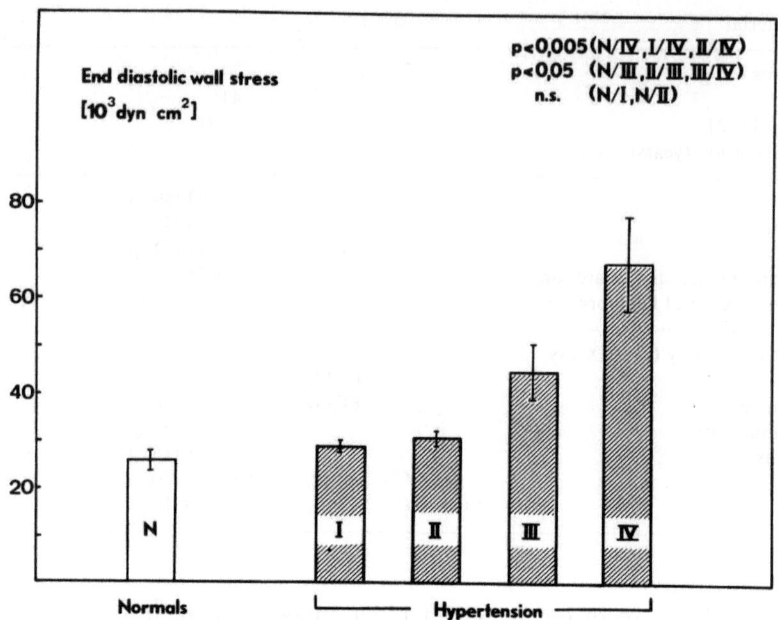

Fig. 29. End-diastolic wall stresses in the hypertension groups investigated

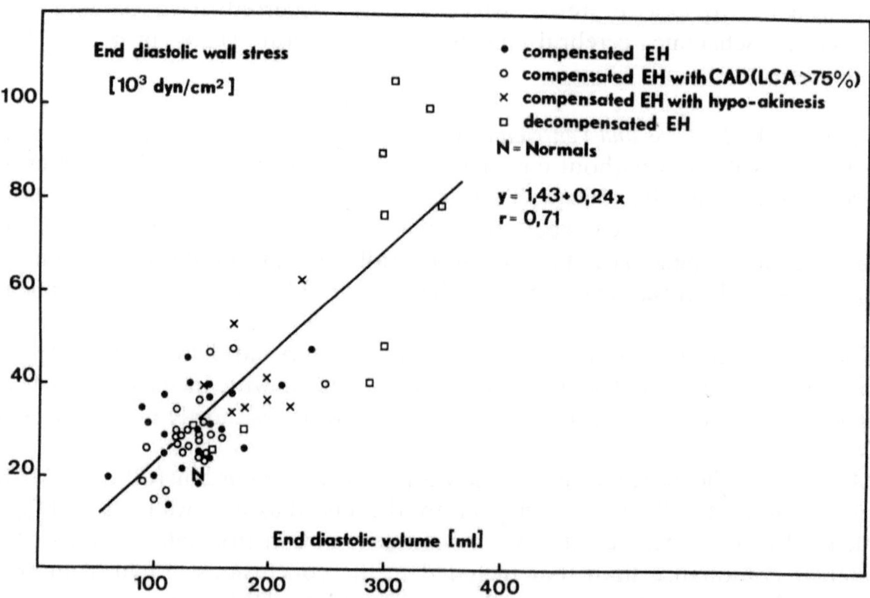

Fig. 30. Relationship between end-diastolic volume and end-diastolic wall stress of the left ventricle. To simplify matters the relationship between the two variables was assumed to be linear

tension with and without coronary stenoses, whereas in patients with hypertension and regional wall contraction disturbances as well as in those with decompensated hypertension it appears to be markedly reduced. This means that despite significant left ventricular hypertrophy (compensated hypertensives with and without coronary stenoses) ventricular compliance can be largely normal. Therefore, in essential hypertension significant losses in compliance become apparent only following secondary heart diseases (hypokinesis, akinesis) and in the decompensated stage of hypertension. The inclusion of mass-volume ratio, volume to mass ratio and wall thickness-radius ratio, which are already partly allowed for in the LMFS index, did not contribute to any further differentiation of the groups.

Systolic Wall Stress and Degree of Hypertrophy. The peak circumferential wall stress of the left ventricle — i. e. both the ventricular total stress and the wall stress that, in addition to the end-diastolic wall stress, was maximally and actively developed by the left ventricle during systole — showed normal mean values in compensated hypertensives with and without coronary stenoses (Table 11). However, in

Table 10. Diastolic wall stress and compliance indices of the left ventricle. Group I: compensated essential hypertension without coronary stenoses; group II: compensated essential hypertension with coronary stenoses (LCA > 75%); group III: compensated essential hypertension with regional wall contraction disturbances (hypo- and akinesis); group IV: decompensated essential hypertension

| | Normotension | \multicolumn{4}{c}{Essential Hypertension} | | | |
		I	II	III	IV
T_{diast} [10^3 dyn/cm^2]	26 ± 3	28 ± 2	31 ± 6	44 $\pm 6^*$	68 $\pm 10^{**}$
dp/dV [mm Hg/ml]	0.151 ± 0.008	0.162 ± 0.011	0.213 ± 0.016	0.326 ± 0.019	0.55 ± 0.032
dV/dp [ml/mm Hg]	6.78 ± 1.02	6.12 ± 0.92	4.8 ± 0.57	3.12 ± 0.21	1.81 $\pm 0.10^*$
dV/dp $\cdot$ V [l/mm Hg]	0.079 ± 0.009	0.077 ± 0.010	0.057 $\pm 0.006^*$	0.029 $\pm 0.001^{**}$	0.011 $\pm 0.001^{**}$
LMFS (rel. units)	508 ± 98	582 ± 72	623 ± 119	1120 $\pm 223^{**}$	1610 $\pm 204^{**}$

$$LMSF = T_{diast} \cdot \left(\frac{dV \cdot d}{3V \cdot dP} \right) \quad * \; p < 0.01 \quad ** \; p < 0.005$$

Table 11. End-diastolic and systolic wall stresses of the left ventricle. The tension-time index of the left ventricle is to be regarded as the product of peak systolic wall stress (T_{syst}) and heart rate. The ventricular performance is the product of peak systolic wall stress (T_{syst}) and stroke index. For level of significance, see Figs. 29 and 32

| | Normotension | \multicolumn{4}{c}{Essential Hypertension} | | | |
		I	II	III	IV
T_{diast} [10^3 dyn/cm^2]	26 ± 3	28 ± 2	31 ± 6	44 ± 6	68 ± 10
T_{syst} [10^3 dyn/cm^2]	220 ± 9	232 ± 8	208 ± 19	256 ± 18	369 ± 26
T_{ges} [10^3 dyn/cm^2]	246 ± 11	260 ± 9	239 ± 14	300 ± 17	437 ± 23
T_{syst}/T_{diast}	8.46	8.28	6.71	5.81	5.43
$T_{syst} \cdot n$ [10^3 dyn/cm$^2 \cdot$ min]	16 280	17 169	16 224	21 456	28 782
$T_{syst} \cdot$ SVI (rel. units)	11 220	11 600	10 192	10 496	14 760

hypertensives with regional wall contraction disturbances the peak systolic wall stress increased slightly, and in patients with decompensated hypertension a considerable rise was observed. In relation to end-diastolic wall stress the maximal rise in wall stress during systole was found to be almost similar for normotensives and compensated hypertensives without coronary stenoses, whereas the relationship between peak systolic and end-diastolic wall stress decreased in proportion to the increasing coronary and myocardial secondary diseases of essential hypertension (Table 11). This is likely to indicate that — with comparable arterial pressure load — a higher diastolic wall stress and a greater increase in preload are required in order to ensure high systolic wall stress in patients with decompensated essential hypertension than in patients with compensated hypertension.

Parallel to the increasing diastolic and systolic wall stress there was an increase in that index which is the product of peak systolic wall stress and heart rate and which serves as a correlate to the systolic tension-time index. Thus, in patients suffering from coronary diseases plus hypertension with regional wall contraction disturbances (group III) this index exceeded normal value by 32%, and in patients with compensated hypertension, by 77%. Under similar heart rate conditions the changes in direction of the tension-frequency product are therefore in line with the changes in percentage of the peak systolic wall stress so that neither different nor elucidative statements were achieved by this. It was, however, striking that maximal ventricular performance, which is calculated as the product of peak systolic wall stress (afterload) and stroke index, was highest in patients with decompensated hypertension, exceeding normal levels by 32%. Maximal performance of the ventricle was therefore seen in that hypertension group in which the forward pumping function was lowest as indicated by a fall in cardiac index, stroke index and ejection fraction (Table 11). Hence, there appears to be a considerable disproportion between 'internal' ventricular performance and external cardiac work of the dilated ventricles in patients suffering from decompensated hypertension.

The end-diastolic and peak systolic wall stresses decreased with increasing mass-volume ratio of the left ventricle (Figs. 31–33). Here, hypertensives with increased mass-volume ratio and normal or lowered diastolic or systolic wall stress may approach towards the abscissas a control group with hypertrophic obstructive cardiomyopathy and hypertensives with almost normal mass-volume ratios and increased diastolic and systolic wall stresses approach towards the coordinates a control group with decompensated aortic vitia in the upper part. Taking the normal range as a basis, wall stresses may on the one hand decrease with an increasing mass-volume ratio and increase with a decreasing mass-volume ratio; on the other hand, despite a comparable increase in absolute left ventricular mass, normal, lowered and increased wall stresses are obtained in essential hypertension as a result of changes in the cavum of the ventricle and hence in the ventricular radius. To assess the *proportionality of hypertrophy* in essential hypertension, not only the muscle mass but also the intraventricular volume, which varies from patient to patient, and the wall stress have to be taken into consideration. As far as form is concerned, similar relationships were seen when taking the wall thickness-radius ratio as the basis of mass-volume ratio (Figs. 34, 35).

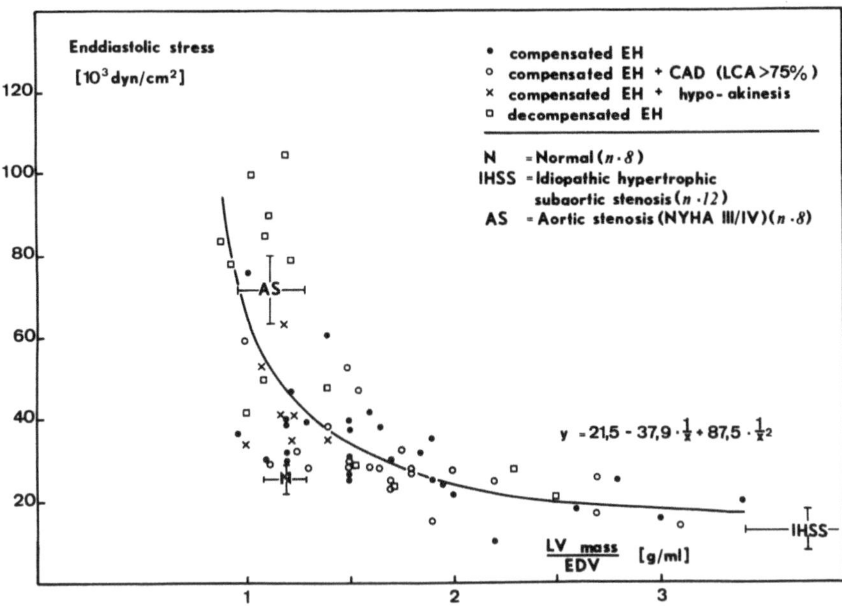

Fig. 31. The relationship between mass-volume ratio of the left ventricle and end-diastolic wall stress

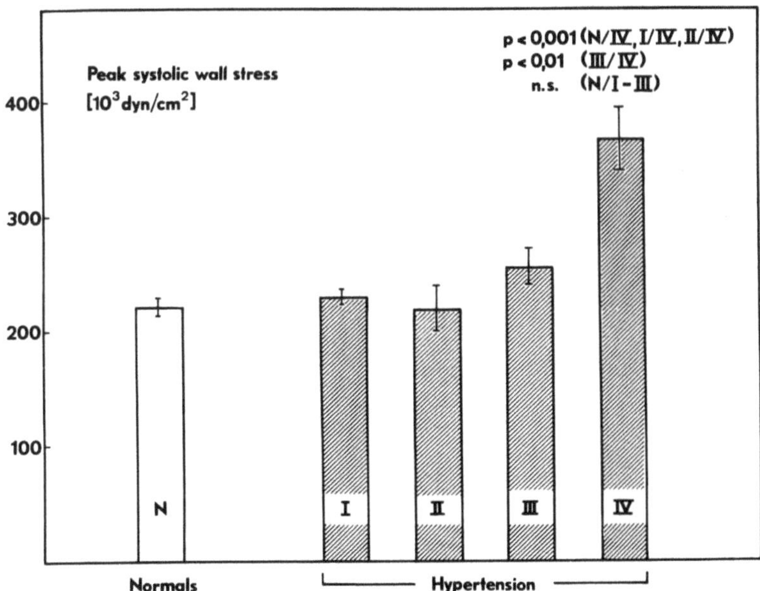

Fig. 32. Peak systolic wall stresses in the hypertension groups investigated

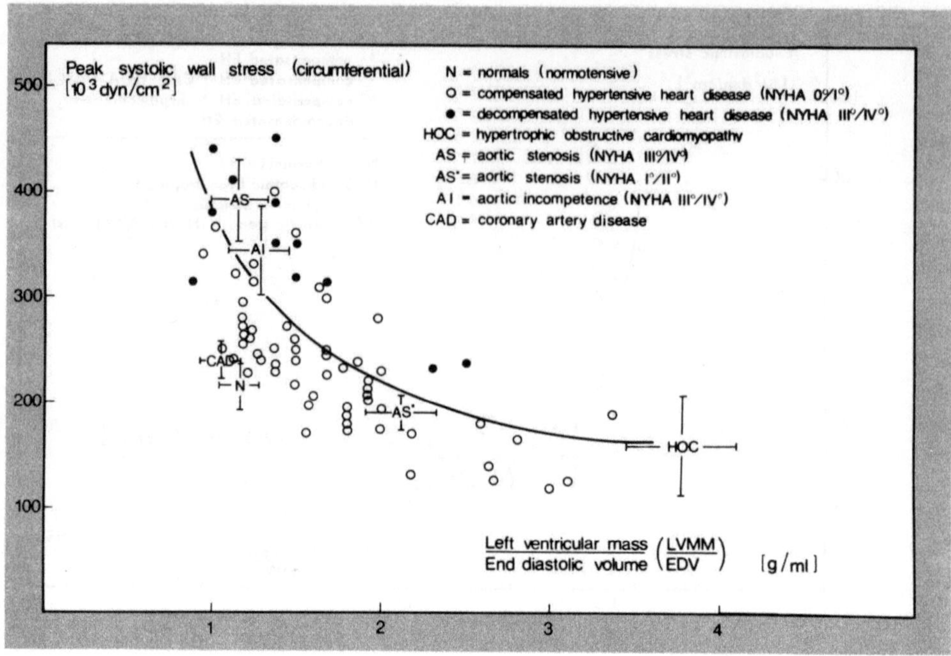

Fig. 33. The relationship between mass-volume ratio of the left ventricle and peak systolic wall stress

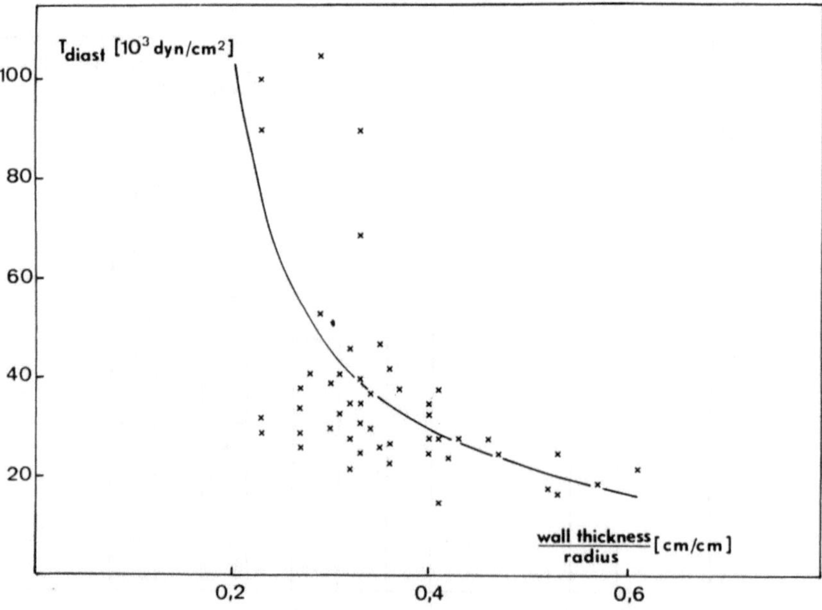

Fig. 34. The relationship between wall thickness-radius ratio of the left ventricle and end-diastolic wall stress

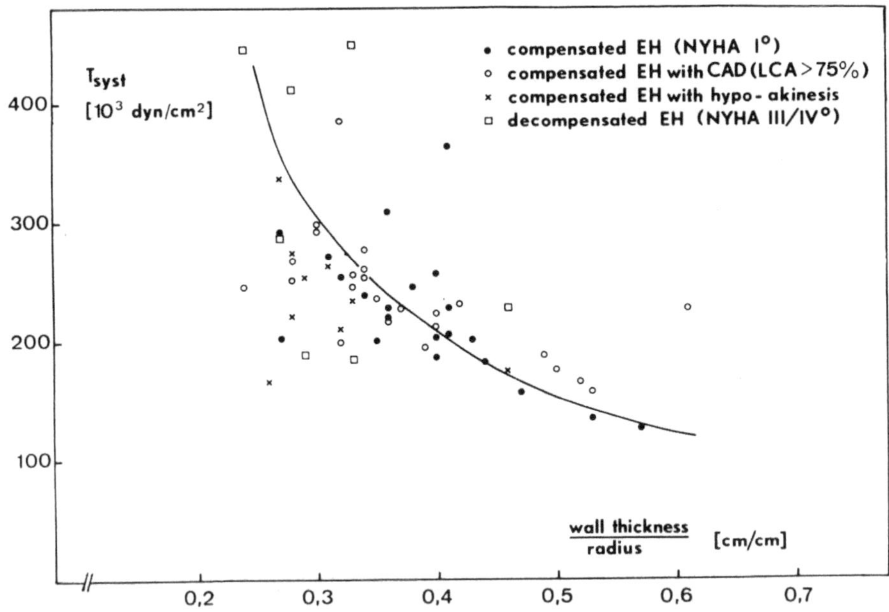

Fig. 35. The relationship between wall thickness-radius ratio and peak systolic wall stress of the left ventricle

Discussion of the Results

From these investigations changes in end-diastolic wall stress, diastolic ventricular compliance and systolic ventricular function became evident during the course of essential hypertension. The decrease in end-diastolic wall stress parallel to an increasing mass-volume ratio illustrates that hypertrophy per se does not necessarily imply a decrease in diastolic compliance even if progressive hypertrophy is almost regularly accompanied by an upswing in diastolic pressure-volume ratio towards higher filling pressures and/or by a steeper rise in pressure-volume ratio [11, 103, 104]. However, this change in pressure-volume ratio is not equivalent to a change in compliance which coincides with a change in myocardial elasticity. Assuming the size of the ventricle to be normal, increasing hypertrophy of the ventricle will be associated with increases in wall thickness and mass and hence an increase in mass-volume ratio. The increase in wall thickness itself could suffice for the end-diastolic wall stress to be kept at a normal or nearly normal level in the presence of constant ventricular radius and unchanged or increasing end-diastolic ventricular pressure. Uncomplicated hypertrophy following essential hypertension may therefore also coincide with a considerable increase in left ventricular mass with normal compliance. This assumption is supported by the fact that compliance indices were seen to be normal in compensated essential hypertensives without coronary stenoses. This means that compliance is not only determined by wall thickness or ventricular mass [33] but above all by mass-volume and wall thickness-radius ratios, and this further means that in uncomplicated compensated essential hypertension compliance can be classified as normal even if severe hypertrophy is present.

Unlike patients suffering from uncomplicated essential hypertension, hypertension groups with coronary artery disease (hypo-, akinesis) and with cardiac decompensation showed a marked decrease in compliance. Parallel to this, a decrease in mass-volume ratio and an increase in end-diastolic wall stress took place. Changes in myocardial structure, being the basis of coronary artery disease, are considered to be the responsible factors so that the decrease in compliance in essential hypertensives with coronary artery disease is predominantly determined by the change in compliance following coronary manifestation [102, 106], Here again, the hypertrophic factor seems to be of secondary importance. In compensated hypertensives on the other hand, in whom end-diastolic pressure and volume rise considerably, an effective inclusion of the preload and a preload-related decrease in compliance cannot be excluded. This view is supported by the behaviour shown by wall stresses and examined compliance indices, indicating that the rise in preload increases with increasing haemodynamic severity. However, in this connection one has to bear in mind that the end-diastolic wall stress rises with decreasing mass-volume ratio for reasons of ventricular geometry only. Since a decrease in mass-volume ratio is mostly associated with ventricular dilatation, the enlarged ventricular radius and the relative decrease in wall thickness always produce changes in those compliance indices in which these parameters are included mathematically. Therefore the possibility of obtaining information on the actual preload by means of these indices is limited, even though relevant indices, e. g. LMFS, lg dP/dV, are used to determine the compliance of the myocardium [27–29, 62].

Because of the inclusion of the Frank-Starling mechanism, effective increase in the preload should be associated with an increase in the pumping function of the left ventricle. This is how in essential hypertension the decrease in contractility, which develops with increasing haemodynamic severity, could be compensated. Apart from the ejection fraction, parameters for the determination of the pumping function would be those which are largely independent of or little influenced by the contractility, such as pressure-volume performance and tension-time index. Here only parameters of the ventricular function are relevant since with the effective forward parameters no allowance is made for the effects of a different ventricular geometry on ventricular performance. Therefore in order to assess ventricular performance, parameters are used which include data on the ability of the ventricle to produce stress and to stimulate volume. Such parameters are above all the wall stress and the products of wall stress and rate or of wall stress and shortening (stroke volume). Peak systolic wall stress and total stress were highest in the hypertensives of groups III and IV. Whereas the end-diastolic wall stress up to group IV increased by 2.62 times the normal value, the peak systolic wall stress only increased by 1.68 times the normal value. Accordingly, the ratio of peak systolic to end-diastolic wall stress was markedly reduced in groups III and IV. Despite comparable arterial pressure load the end-diastolic wall stress thus rises higher with increasing severity of essential hypertension than does systolic wall stress, so that the myocardial preload is likely to increase according to the respective pressure-volume ratio of the ventricle. The parameters of the tension-time index and ventricular performance were likewise increased by between 28% and 67% in the hypertensives of groups III and IV in comparison with decompensated hypertensives. This indicates the inclusion of the Frank-Starling mechanism to be effective but not sufficient in ensuring a normal forward pumping function of the left ventricle, since external cardiac work, cardiac index and stroke index decreased with increasing haemodynamic severity in essential hypertensives. Thus, as far as ventricular performance is concerned, increasing ventricular dilatation and increasing haemodynamic severity lead to a growing disproportion between forward performance and ventricular performance insofar as there is a decrease in peripherally measurable pumping values and an increase in internal cardiac performance and ventricular performance values. Especially in decompensated essential hypertension the latter becomes evident in the form of a marked rise in peak systolic wall stress and ventricular performance, which must be regarded as the major determinants of myocardial energy requirements.

The shown relations between wall stress, diastolic compliance and systolic ventricular performance allow the hypertrophied left ventricle in essential hypertension to be quantitatively assessed and diagnostically classified on the basis of degree of hypertrophy and ventricular function. End-diastolic and peak systolic wall stresses of the left ventricle decrease with increasing mass-volume ratio. Ventricular function and compliance are either normal or increased. Left ventricular oxygen consumption per unit of weight is either normal or reduced. X-ray of the heart reveals either a normal size or a moderate enlargement of the left ventricle, the end-diastolic volume is either normal or reduced during considerable increase in wall thickness and the ejection fraction is normal. However, 14% of these patients are expected to develop asymmetric or irregular ventricular wall hypertrophy. On the other hand, end-diastolic and systolic wall stresses increase with decreasing mass-volume ratio. There will be a simultaneous decrease in ventricular compliance and ventricular function (ejection fraction, stroke index, cardiac index etc.). Internal ventricular performance, calculated as the product of peak wall stress and stroke index, is markedly increased, so that a growing discrepancy develops between the effective forward pumping performance and ventricular performance to the disadvantage of the effective forward pumping performance. Since systolic and total *wall stresses* of the left ventricle are the decisive determinants of *myocardial oxygen consumption*, the myocardial oxygen demand will be increased in these patients. Thus, there is an increased susceptibility to ischaemia, especially in the presence of secondary coronary diseases.

Therefore, these investigations show that increasing haemodynamic severity during essential hypertension is characterized by a decrease in mass-volume ratio, increases in ventricular wall stress and internal ventricular performance, decreases in ventricular compliance and function, and an increase in myocardial energy requirements (Fig. 36). As to the clinicopractical measures for diagnosing and quantifying hypertensive heart diseases, it has to be stated that a decrease in mass-volume ratio of the hypertensive heart which inhibits the function of the ventricle is almost always associated with an increase in left ventricular size and cardiac dilatation. The latter is therefore the simplest criterion for establishing the presence of a developing or progressing heart disease.

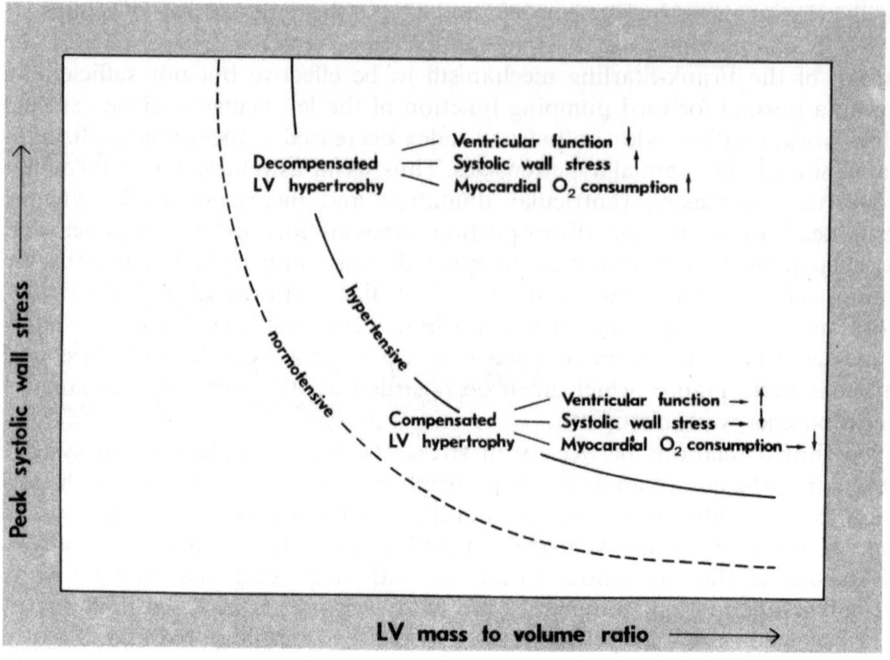

Fig. 36. Diagnostic classification of the hypertension groups on the basis of degree of hypertension (mass-volume ratio) and wall stress. Note the dependence of left ventricular function and energy demand on the degree of hypertrophy and systolic wall stress

3.5 Stress and Function

Results

With an increase in systolic wall stress, a decrease in cardiac function occurred. Patients with the largest wall stress (Fig. 37) (decompensated essential hypertension, group IV) had the lowest ejection fraction and lowest ejection phase indices. A similar relationship was also present for chronic hypertrophic heart disease of various origin (Fig. 38). Since systolic wall stress represents the major determinant of the left ventricular afterload, an *afterload-dependent decrease in left ventricular function* is thereby demonstrated. It may be assumed that the decrease in function parallel with the increase in heart size or in end-diastolic volume (see Fig. 6) depends on the augmentation of wall stress parallel with an increase in end-diastolic volume. It may be further assumed that this relationship — except for wall stress — depends on the *contractile state* of the myocardium. Parallel with an increase in contractility, an increase in left ventricular function at equal wall stress (i.e. at equal afterload) may occur (Fig. 39); alternatively, negatively inotropic interventions may depress ventricular function without an increase in systolic wall-stress.

The close relationship between stress and function becomes evident also for normotensive or hypertensive *hypertrophic heart disease* on the basis of coronary or valvular lesions (Table 12). Likewise the increase in myocardial energy demand parallel with stress increase can be shown for this large group of patients with left ventricular overload.

56

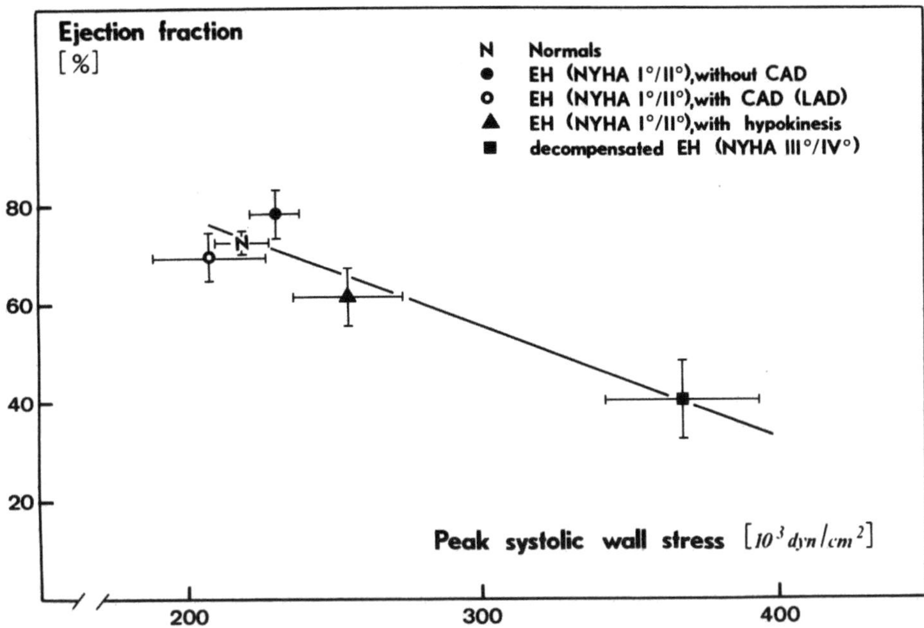

Fig. 37. Relationship between peak systolic wall stress and ventricular function in hypertensive heart disease as expressed by the LV ejection fraction (total stroke volume divided by end-diastolic volume). Note the inverse relationship, i.e. the decrease in function with increase in wall stress

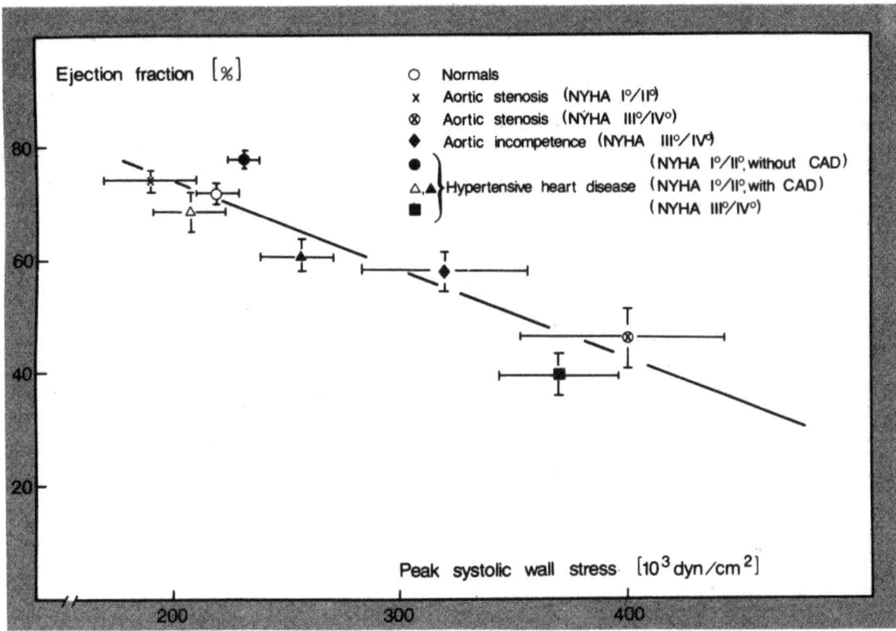

Fig. 38. Relationship between peak systolic wall stress and ventricular function, as expressed by the LV ejection fraction, in hypertrophic heart disease of various origin. Note the decrease in function with increase in wall stress

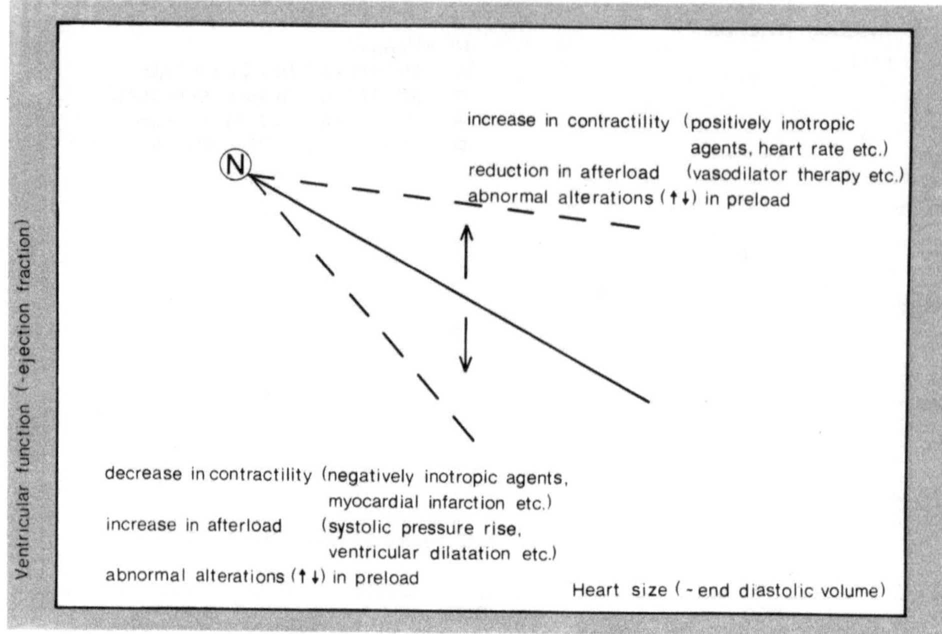

Fig. 39. Schematic representation of the relationships between left ventricular end-diastolic volume ($\sim$ heart size) and left ventricular function (*ordinate*). The steepness of regression presumably may be modified by inotropic interventions, by changes in preload and by changes in afterload (systolic wall stress)

Table 12. Ejection fraction, left ventricular (LV) mass, mass-volume ratio, peak systolic wall stress (T_{syst}), myocardial oxygen consumption ($M\dot{V}O_2$) and total left ventricular oxygen consumption ($L\dot{V}O_2$) in normals (normotensive, non-hypertrophied) and in various diseases of the heart. CAD, coronary artery disease; SVD, small vessel disease, on the basis of coronary and systemic immune complex vasculitis; AS, aortic stenosis; AI, aortic incompetence; HOC, hypertrophic obstructive cardiomyopathy; EH, essential hypertension; MI, mitral incompetence; MV, combined mitral valve lesions. Note the increase in myocardial oxygen consumption per weight unit ($M\dot{V}O_2$) with an increase in wall stress; note further the decrease in LV function (EF) with an increase in systolic wall stress

	N =	Ejection fraction [%]	LV mass [g/m²]	LV mass to volume ratio [g/ml]	T_{syst} [10³ dyn/cm²]	$M\dot{V}O_2$ [ml/min · 100 G]	$L\dot{V}O_2$ [ml/min]
Normals	12	72± 2	92± 6	1.21±0.12	220± 9	7.98±0.52	13.3±2.1
CAD	36	52±11	145±22ˣ	1.12±0.16	236±18	7.9 ±0.39	20.6±3.2
SVD	8	69± 8	84±14	1.18±0.21	206±22	6.4 ±0.6ˣ	9.7±0.91ˣ
AS*	6	74± 4	145±10ˣˣ	2.1 ±0.31	192±23	8.1 ±0.8	21.1±2.3ˣˣ
AS**	9	46±11	190±17●	1.01±0.11	396±95ˣˣ	14.9 ±1.6●	51.0±6.9●
AI	12	58± 7	174±22●	1.12±0.13	329±36ˣ	14.2 ±1.4●	45.4±4.7●
HOC	12	78± 6	~ 228	~ 3.78	142±52	8.6 ±1.21	35.3±3.6
EH	92	62± 6	152±12●	1.52±0.33	266±18ˣˣ	10.7 ±0.38●	29.3±4.1●
MI	20	63± 9	132±11ˣ	1.19±0.09	267±11ˣ	9.82±0.21ˣˣ	21.6±0.92
MV	44	62±12	149± 9ˣˣ	1.20±0.10	248±32ˣ	9.22±0.99ˣ	24.9±2.9ˣ

AS* : Clinically compensated (NYHA I●/II●), concentric hypertrophy
AS**: Clinically decompensated (NYHA III●/IV●), LV dilatation
ˣ p < 0,05   ˣˣ p < 0,01   ● p < 0,001

Discussion of the Results

Therapeutic Implications. Relating to the *intrinsic relationship between mass-volume ratio and systolic wall stress* (see Fig. 33), the influence of therapeutic interventions in the course of hypertensive or non-hypertensive hypertrophic heart disease may be evaluated (Fig. 40): (1) Reduction in afterload (A → B) results in marked reduction in systolic wall stress. Stress reduction is greater in a dilated than in a non-dilated heart. (2) Reduction in preload (A → C) results in marked change in the mass-volume ratio with however, only moderate decrease in systolic wall stress. (3) Finally, reductions in both preload and afterload lead to most pronounced stress alterations (A → D). Alternatively, increases in preload, in afterload or in both preload and afterload are associated with comparable increases in systolic wall stress.

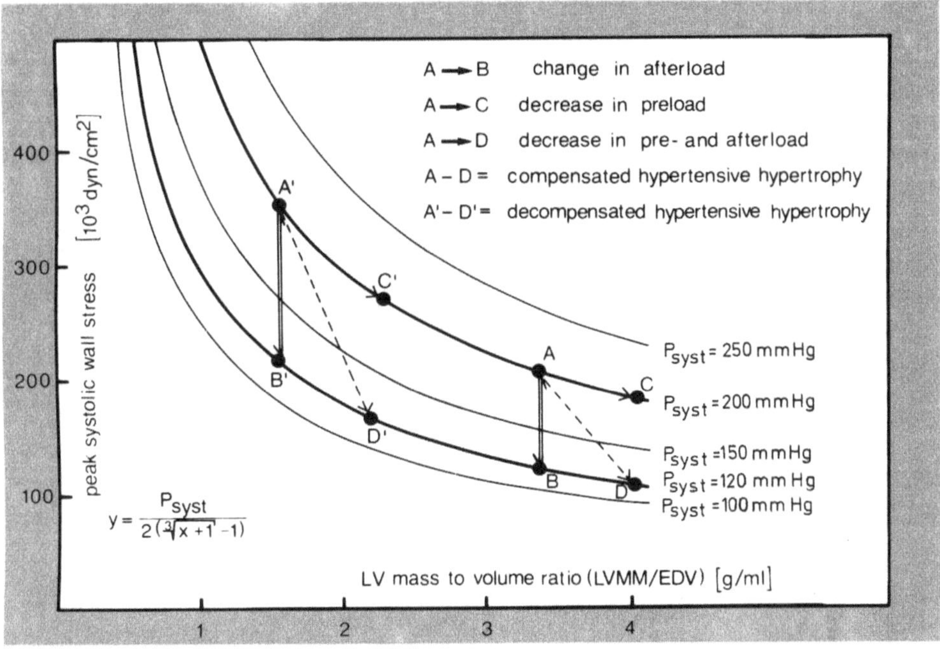

Fig. 40. Diagrammatic representation of the relationships between the mass-volume ratio (*abscissa*) and peak systolic wall stress (*ordinate*) for different isobaric conditions (original data, see Table 12). Calculation of isobares was performed by use of the Laplace equation. The non-linearity of these isobaric relationships implies that systolic pressure changes at an initially high mass-volume ratio have lower stress changes than the same systolic pressure changes at a low mass-volume ratio: an equal systolic pressure rise, e. g. from 120 mm Hg to 200 mm Hg (i. e. from B to A) at a mass-volume ratio of 3.5 leads to stress increase of only 80 units (10^3 dyn/cm²). However, the same pressure rise (i. e. from B' to A') at a mass-volume ratio of 1.5 results in a considerable increase in systolic wall stress by 160 units. The same consequences are valid for therapeutically induced pressure reductions (from A' to B' and from A to B, respectively). This means that systolic pressure increase in dilated hypertensive heart disease leads to greater increase in stress and myocardial energy demand than the same pressure increase in a non-dilated heart. Conversely, systolic and metabolic unloading of the left ventricle at equal pressure reduction is greater or more effective in a dilated than in a non-dilated heart. Thus, the relationship between mass-volume ratio and stress elucidates the importance of heart size and systolic wall stress in changes in stress and hence in ventricular function and myocardial energy demand

Pressure-Induced Stress Alterations and $M\dot{V}O_2$. An increase (hypertensive crisis) or decrease (antihypertensive treatment) in systolic pressure is associated with alterations in systolic wall stress and, hence, in $M\dot{V}O_2$. However, pressure-induced stress alterations depend on the individual isobaric conditions as well as on the initial mass-volume ratio (Fig. 41). An equal rise in pressure (e. g. from 120 to 200 mm Hg) (A′→ B′) at a mass-volume ratio of 4 g/ml leads to a stress increase of only 80×10^3 dyn/cm^2, whereas the same rise in pressure (A → B) at a mass-volume ratio of 1.2 is followed by a considerable increase in stress of 180×10^3 dyn/cm^2. The same calculations and consequences as to systolic stress and, hence, $M\dot{V}O_2$ are valid for therapeutically induced pressure reductions (see legend to Fig. 40). This means that from a diagnostic and prognostic point of view, a rise in systolic pressure in a *dilated* hypertensive heart causes a greater increase in peak systolic wall stress and in $M\dot{V}O_2$ than the same pressure increase in a *non-dilated*, hypertensive heart. Because both stress and metabolic reserves are limited in man, the left ventricular stress capacity is increasingly reduced with: (1) an *increase in initial systolic stress*, (2) a *decrease in mass-volume ratio*, and (3) *an increase in systolic pressure*. However, a therapeutic reduction in systolic pressure will lead to greater reduction in both stress and oxygen consumption in patients with left ventricular dilatation than in patients with concentric hypertrophy (Fig. 41). Thus, the relationship between mass-volume ratio and peak systolic wall stress elucidates the importance of

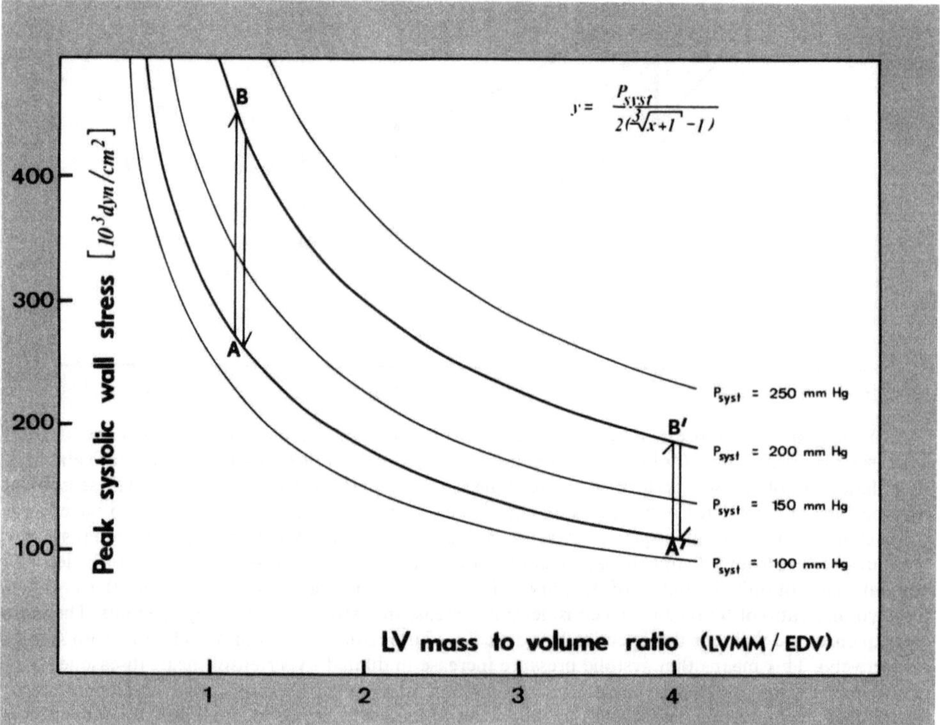

Fig. 41. Relationship between left ventricular (LV) mass-volume ratio (LVMM/EDV) (x) and peak systolic wall stress (y) at different isobaric conditions. P$_{syst}$ peak systolic pressure

60

pressure-dependent changes in systolic stress and, hence, in myocardial stress and metabolic reserve.

Systolic Stress Reserve. With regard to previous measurements in isolated human left ventricular myocardium, the maximum isometric tension development (preload at L_{max}) which can be achieved by human heart muscle averages 5–6 g/mm^2. When expressed in dyn/cm^2, maximum stress values of 500–600 (10^3 dyn/cm^2) (T_{max}) ought to be expected. The ratio of T_{max} to instantaneous T_{syst} (T_{max}/T_{syst} = systolic stress reserve) depends on both the instantaneous T_{syst} (as influenced by systolic pressure, mass and volume) and the amount of T_{max} (as influenced by inotropic interventions and heart rate) (Figs. 42, 43). Provided that T_{max} is quantitatively comparable in different stages of chronic hypertrophy, it may be assumed that low initial stress, as in concentric hypertrophy with large mass-volume ratio, has large stress reserve and that the latter is reduced at high initial stress (as in chronic LV dilatation). T_{max}/T_{syst} therefore may be improved by lowering instantaneous T_{syst} or by increasing T_{max}.

It may be concluded from these results that determination of LV wall dynamics, of coronary blood flow and of oxygen consumption provides useful basis for the evaluation of the *degree of LV hypertrophy* and of myocardial energy demand in chronic hypertrophic heart disease.

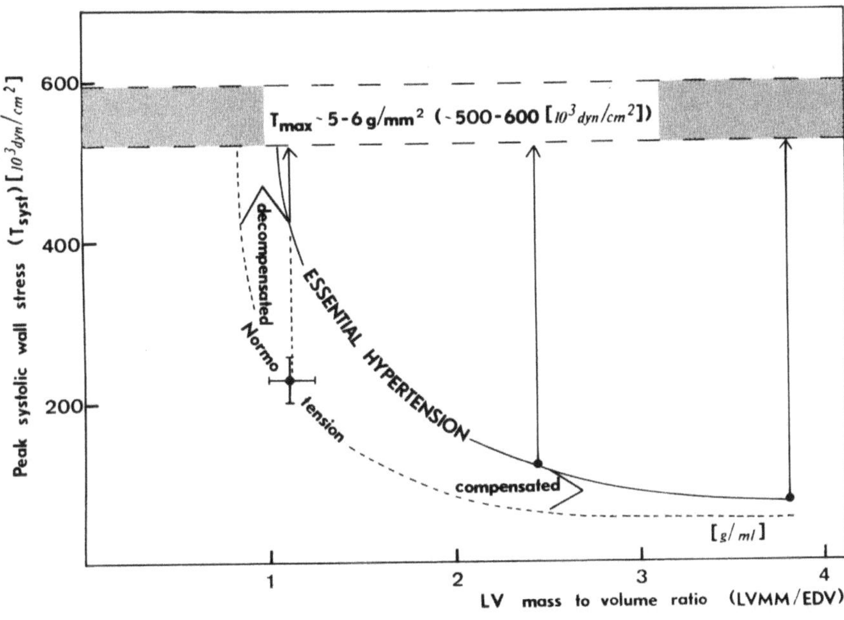

Fig. 42. Relationship between mass-volume ratio (*abscissa*) and peak systolic wall stress (*ordinate*) for non-hypertensives and hypertensives. Decompensated heart disease has a normal or decreased mass-volume ratio, but an increased systolic wall stress; compensated hypertensive heart disease has a normal or increased mass-volume ratio and normal or reduced systolic wall stress. Maximum systolic wall stress of the human heart, which presumably may be developed under maximum load, is defined as T_{max}. Value of 5–6 g/mm^2 has been transferred from data of maximum stress development of isolated human ventricular myocardium. The ratio of instantaneous to maximum stress, i.e. systolic stress reserve, is larger in compensated than in decompensated heart disease (*vertical arrows*)

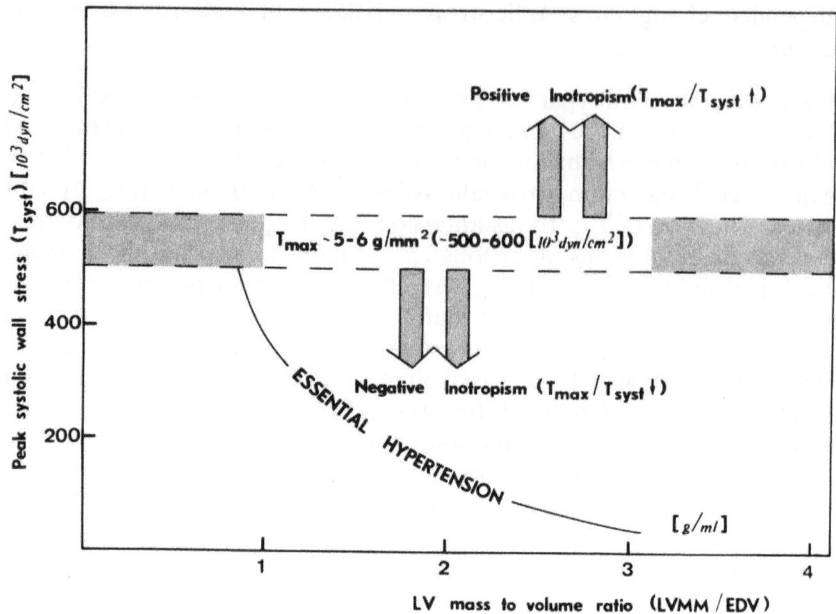

Fig. 43. Influence of inotropic interventions on maximum systolic stress development and systolic stress reserve

3.6 Ventricular Mass, Wall Stress and Degree of Hypertrophy: Diagnostic and Therapeutic Consequences

The aim of this section is to analyse the findings among patients with essential hypertension with respect to the *degree of hypertrophy* or the proportionality of hypertrophy, which are influenced by the relationships between systolic pressure, ventricular mass, intraventricular volume and resultant wall stress. Diagnostic possibilities and therapeutic consequences should especially be derived from the degree of left ventricular pressure load and the degree of ventricular hypertrophy. For comparative purposes the findings on ventricular dynamics and the degree of hypertrophy from animal experiments (spontaneously hypertensive rats) are made available.

These investigations were performed (1) in 64 patients with essential hypertension in the course of diagnostic cardiac catheterisation, coronary angiography and ventriculography, (2) in animal experiments involving spontaneously hypertensive and cardially compensated rats (9–21 weeks old, Okamoto/Aoki strain). Methodological details have already been made available [11, 12, 67]. Evaluation of the data was performed for those patients in whom intraventricular pressure and volume were measured and in whom ventricular mass, mass-volume ratio and peak systolic wall stress were assessed by means of quantitative ventriculography.

62

Case Material. Of the 64 patients, 31 suffered from compensated hypertension without coronary stenoses, 16 had compensated hypertension with significant coronary stenoses, 9 had compensated hypertension with regional wall contraction disturbances (hypo-, akinesis) and 8 suffered from decompensated hypertension. The intraventricular pressure measured in the course of invaside diagnostics showed a minimal systolic value of 156 mm Hg and a peak systolic value of 295 mm Hg (Fig. 44). Here, the peak systolic circumferential wall stresses (T_{syst}) achieved were between 100 and 450 (10^3 dyn/cm^2). Thus, systolic ventricular pressure and T_{syst} varied by factors of 1.9 and 4.5 respectively. From this it becomes evident that in *all* hypertensives ventricular geometry (wall thickness, radius or muscle mass, intraventricular volume) changes by at least twice normal, since a change in pressure alone will not be sufficient to induce a change in wall stress by 4.5 times.

Degree of Hypertrophy and Proportionality of Hypertrophy. Provided that proportional hypertrophy is present there will be an increase in mass-volume ratio with increasing pressure load since the increase in wall thickness or muscle mass normally exceeds the increase in intraventricular volume in compensated and harmoniously hypertrophied essential hypertension. From the relationship between both variables, i.e. between systolic pressure as *measure* of the pressure load and mass-volume ratio as *resultant* of the pressure load, no directed correlation became evident in the hypertensives investigated (Fig. 44). Considering the different

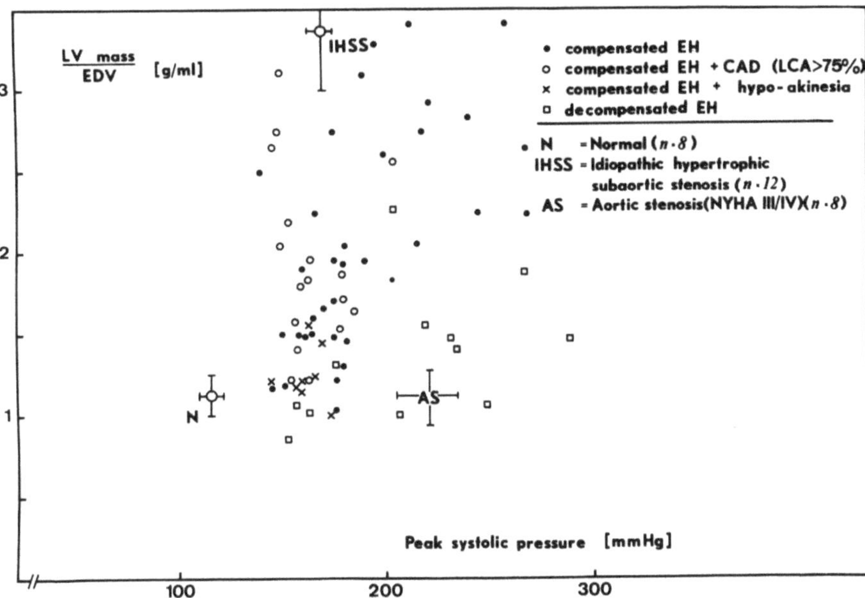

Fig. 44. The relationship between systolic pressure and mass-volume ratio in the hypertensives investigated. Note the missing correlation between the two variables when neglecting the respective isostress ranges (see also Fig. 45)

degrees of hypertrophy, varying in the hypertensives by a factor of more than 3, a comparable change in systolic wall stress could be assumed, since the relationship between intraventricular pressure and mass-volume ratio is determined by the individual systolic wall stress. Accordingly, in essential hypertensives, those who had similar wall stress values were characterised on the basis of non-overlapping ranges (Fig. 45). The spectrum of relationships illustrates that the inclusion of isostress ranges enables the cluster of points to be allocated to the systolic pressure on the one hand, and to the mass-volume ratio on the other (Figs. 45 and 46). When systolic pressure remains level, peak systolic wall stress decreases with increasing mass-volume ratio. In contrast, when the mass-volume ratio remains the same, peak systolic wall stress increases with increasing systolic pressure. However, within the same isostress range, the wall stress can remain unchanged — even during extreme increase — resulting from an increase in mass-volume ratio — as long as there is mutual proportionallity of the relationships between pressure, volume and muscle mass.

During acute pharmacological and haemodynamic interventions, overlappings and shiftings in the function curves of chronic hypertension are likely to occur. From the determination of the relationships between systolic pressure, mass-volume ratio and peak wall stress in the hypertension groups (carried out for reasons of experimental comparison) and from the measurements concerning the

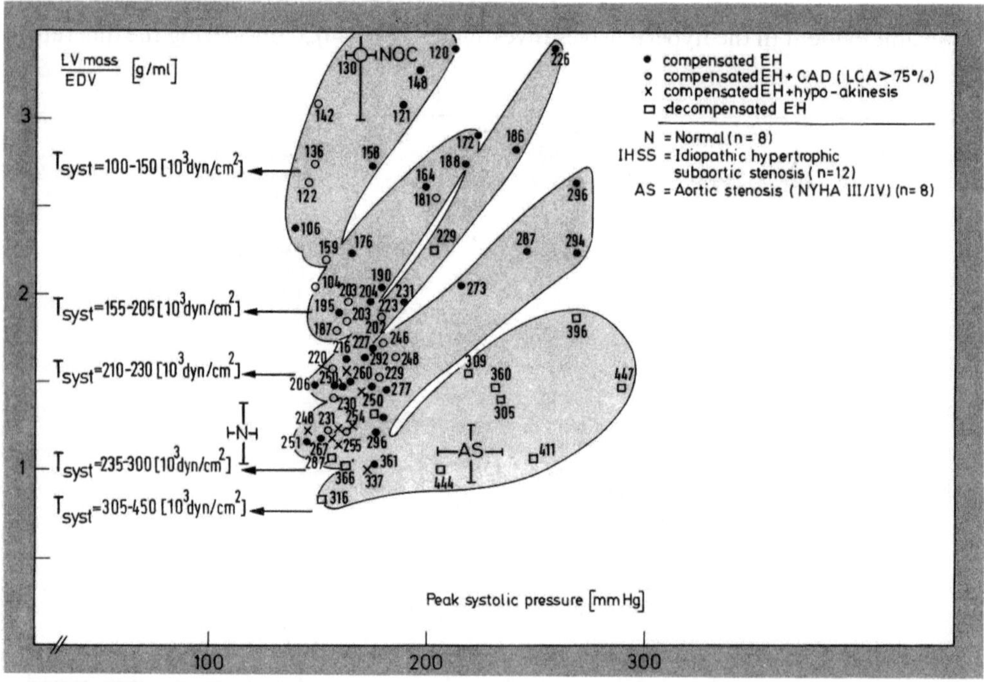

Fig. 45. The relationship between systolic pressure and mass-volume ratio with regard to five isostress ranges formed on the basis of non-overlapping values. Here the same values of essential hypertension were used as in Fig. 44. Note the arrangement of the cluster of points and the satisfactory differentiation of the hypertension groups when references is made to the isostress ranges

applicability of the isostress spectrum, even in the presence of acute interventions on normotensive (NR) and cardially compensated spontaneously hypertensive inbred rats (SHR) (9–21 weeks old), it becomes evident that:

1. Arterial pressure reduction (phlebotomy) coincides with a decrease in systolic wall stress and an increase in wall thickness-radius ratio (analogous to the mass-volume ratio). (Fig. 47).
2. Acute volume load of the left ventricle (infusion) leads to an increase in arterial pressure and a decrease in wall thickness-radius ratio (Fig. 47).
3. Acute left ventricular pressure increase (isovolumetric aortic occlusion) produces considerable ventricular dilatation and an important reduction in wall thickness-radius ratio (Fig. 47).

Peak systolic wall stresses in NRs and SHRs as determined during each function test showed almost similar values despite considerable differences in systolic pressure and wall thickness-radius ratio. This illustrates that in essential hypertension the peak systolic wall stress, i. e. the peak systolic afterload related to the ventricular wall, is kept at almost normal levels by the cardially compensated left ventricle, even in cases of extreme changes in preload and afterload and despite a considerable increase in absolute mass of the left ventricle (+ 80%). Accordingly, in cardially compensated SHRs the degree and proportionality of *hypertrophy* are referred to as *harmonious or adequate since* any change in ventricular working conditions coincides with maintenance of normal peak systolic wall stress. On the other hand, the spectrum of the stress lines reveals that when the wall thickness-

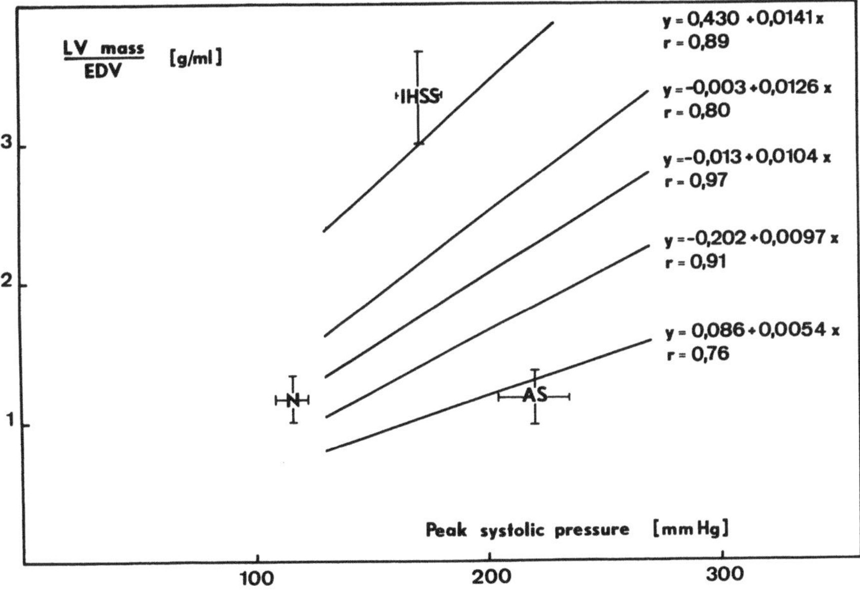

Fig. 46. Regression lines of the relationship between systolic pressure and mass-volume ratio in the essential hypertensives investigated (n = 64). The regression lines were determined according to the isostress ranges (Fig. 45)

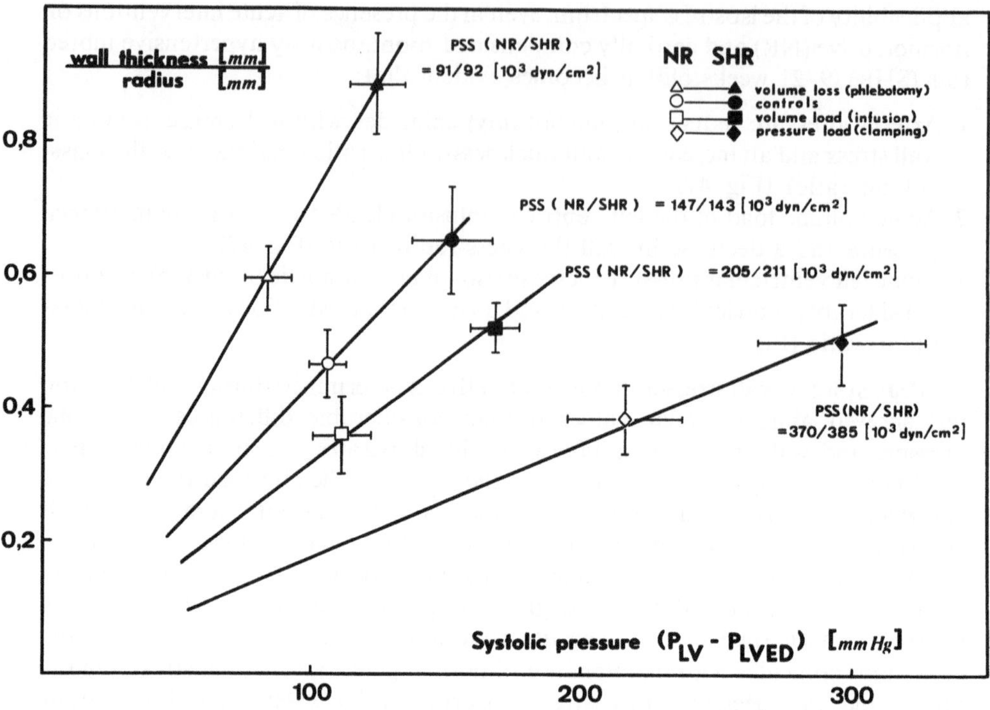

Fig. 47. The relationships between systolic pressure and wall thickness-radius ratio obtained from animal experiments. NR, normotensive rats; SHR, spontaneously hypertensive rats. Note that when there is a change in the working conditions of the left ventricle the systolic wall stress (PSS) varies between 91/92 and 370/385 (10^3 dyn/cm²), i.e. four times its value. Note also that the PSS does not differ between NRs and SHRs during the corresponding interventions (phlebotomy, infusion, clamping) so that in rats the hypertrophy of the cardially compensated hypertensive heart can be considered proportional and harmonious [11, 12]

radius ratio remains the same, peak systolic wall stress of the left ventricle increases with increasing systolic pressure, or that with comparable systolic pressure, peak systolic wall stress also increases with decreasing wall thickness-radius ratio, i.e. with increasing dilatation of the ventricle.

3.7 Reserves of Systolic Wall Stress and Contractility

The contractility reserve of the pressure-loaded left ventricle is primarily determined by its ability to produce and maintain the systolic wall stress. Thus, the contractility reserve is dependent on the systolic wall stress reserve of the left ventricle. The latter in turn may be defined as the relationship of maximal achievable systolic wall stress (T_{max}) to instantaneous systolic wall stress (T_{syst}). In the human heart the maximal achievable systolic wall stress is likely to be about 500–600 (10^3 dyn/cm²) (see Fig. 22, Table 6). This value corresponds to the maximal isometric stress development as measured at the isolated human heart muscle at maximal initial length (L_{max}) (Fig. 48) [93].

With increasing peak systolic wall stress (T_{syst}) and/or decreasing mass-volume ratio, wall stress reserve of the pressure-loaded and hypertrophied left ventricle decreases according to the definition in Fig. 49. In the hypertensive heart, acute peak pressure stresses dependent upon instantaneous systolic wall stress (T_{syst}) thus lead to a decrease in the wall stress reserve with the ventricular dynamic predisposition to produce stress-induced heart failure. During chronic pressure load ventricular hypertrophy follows the corresponding isostress range provided that proportional, i. e. concentric and harmonious, hypertrophy of the myocardium exists, so that the wall stress reserve is allowed to remain unchanged (Fig. 50). Thus, the initial ventricular dynamic situation, as characterised by wall stress reserve and degree of acute pressure loads, determines the function and the contractility reserve of the left ventricle. The systolic wall stress reserve may be improved by positive inotropic interventions (increase in maximal achievable peak systolic wall stress) and by a decrease in arterial pressure (decrease in instantaneous systolic wall stress) (Fig. 51). This enables the left ventricle to produce greater wall stress when there is the same initial ventricular dynamic situation, and to produce a similar increase in wall stress when there is increasing ventricular dilatation with an increase in instantaneous systolic wall stress. Thus, by means of inotropic interventions, e. g. digitalis glycosides, an increase in contractility reserve or left ventricular functional capacity of the dilatating and hypertrophied left ventricle is to be expected in hypertensive heart disease, whereas by means of arterial pressure reduction, e. g. due to beta-

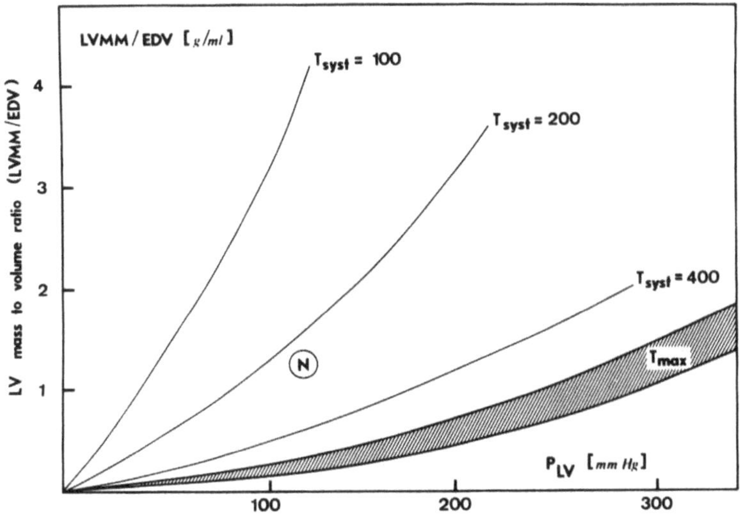

Fig. 48. Schematic diagram of the relationships between systolic pressure in the left ventricle (P_{LV}) and mass-volume ratio with reference to the various isostress ranges of 100, 200 and 400 (10^3 dyn/cm²). The maximal achievable systolic wall stress of the left ventricle (T_{max}) is given in the form of the hatched area on the basis of experimental data from the isolated human ventricular myocardium. *N* normal range. *PLV* systolic pressure in the left ventricle; T_{syst} systolic wall stress; T_{max} maximal achievable systolic wall stress $\cong$ 5–6 g/mm² [~500–600 (10^3 dyn/cm²)]

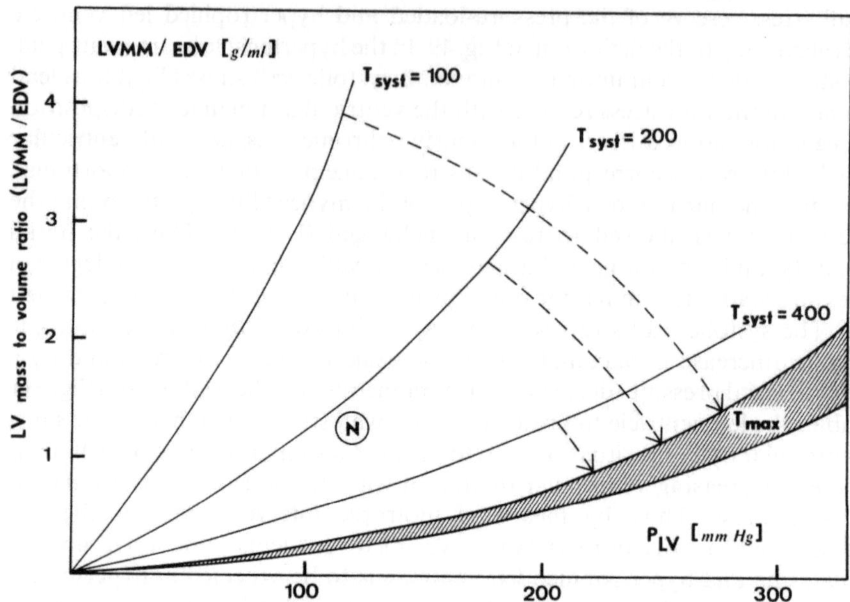

Fig. 49. Schematic diagram of the relationships between systolic pressure in the left ventricle (P_{LV}) and mass-volume ratio. The broken arrows illustrate the wall stress reserve of the left ventricle, being defined as the quotient of the maximal achievable wall stress (T_{max}) to instantaneous wall stress (T_{syst}), i.e. T_{max}/T_{syst}. Note that the wall stress reserve and thus the contractility reserve decrease with increasing initial wall stress i.e. with increasing afterload

receptor blocking agents, a decrease in instantaneous systolic wall stress may lead to an increase in wall stress reserve.

Discussion of the Results

The relationships shown in essential hypertension groups with left ventricular hypertrophy during chronic pressure load and in the hypertrophied left ventricle of SHRs with acute changes in left ventricular working conditions reveal that in equilibrium conditions it is possible by means of the spectrum of stress ranges to define the degree of hypertrophy of the left ventricle in essential hypertension in the presence of both chronic pressure load and acute interventions. The peak systolic *wall stress*, being the resultant of systolic pressure and mass-volume ratio, can be regarded as a clinically useful parameter for the assessment of the *degree of hypertrophy*. There is a significant correlation between systolic wall stress and oxygen consumption of the left ventricle, and there is almost equal quantitative variation of the two parameters throughout the whole range measurable in equilibrium conditions during essential hypertension, so that the systolic wall stress can be regarded as a decisive ventricular dynamic correlate to the energy requirements of the myocardium: hypertensives with *lowered wall stress* reveal,

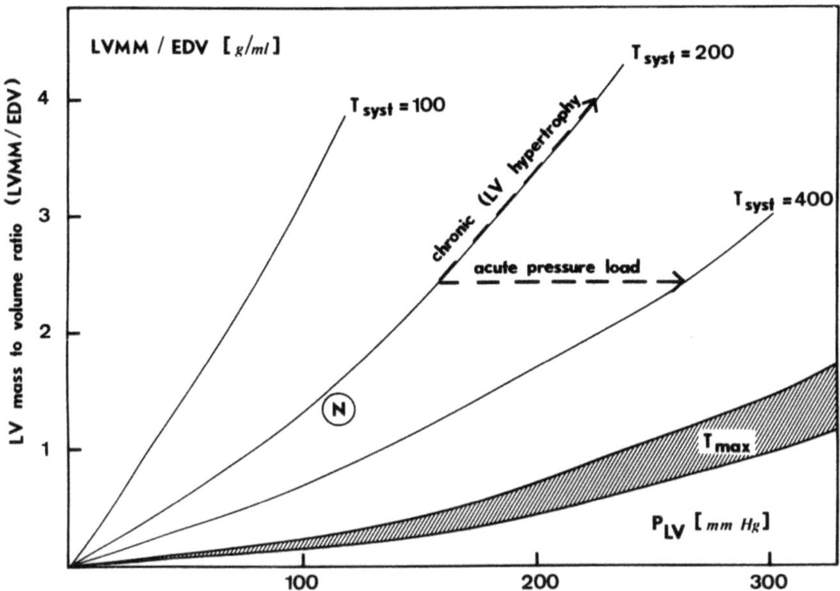

Fig. 50. Schematic diagram of the relationships between systolic pressure in the left ventricle (P_{LV}) and mass-volume ratio during acute and chronic pressure load of the left ventricle. With acute pressure load and almost comparable ventricular dimensions, the increase in systolic wall stress was proportional to the pressure load, so that the wall stress reserve decreases. However, in harmonious and proportional concentric pressure hypertrophy of the left ventricle the isostress range can be maintained so that the systolic wall stress and thus the wall stress reserve remain unchanged

while having a similar systolic pressure, inadequate, i.e. over-proportional, hypertrophy, which favours an increase in mass-volume ratio (Fig. 52). Hypertensives with *normal wall stress* can be classified as proportionally hypertrophied throughout the whole range of arterial pressure and mass-volume ratio. Hypertensives with *raised wall stress* on the other hand, reveal, while having a stable systolic pressure, inadequate, i.e. under-proportional, hypertrophy to the disavantage of a normal mass-volume ratio.

The shown relationships may contribute to the diagnostic classification and differential therapy of essential hypertension from the standpoint of ventricular function and coronary haemodynamics. Hypertensives with high wall stress and normal or lowered mass-volume ratio will be especially predisposed to cardiac risks. The ventricular function is reduced, the myocardial oxygen consumption, increased (Fig. 53). Hypertensives with normal wall stress show normal ventricular function and normal myocardial oxygen consumption in the presence of proportional hypertrophy. Hypertensives with lowered wall stress and high mass-volume ratio show normal or increased ventricular function and normal or reduced myocardial oxygen consumption. Therefore, in essential hypertension, ventricular function and coronary haemodynamics are largely determined by the degree and proportionality of hypertrophy.

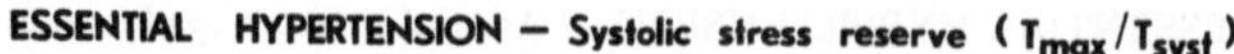

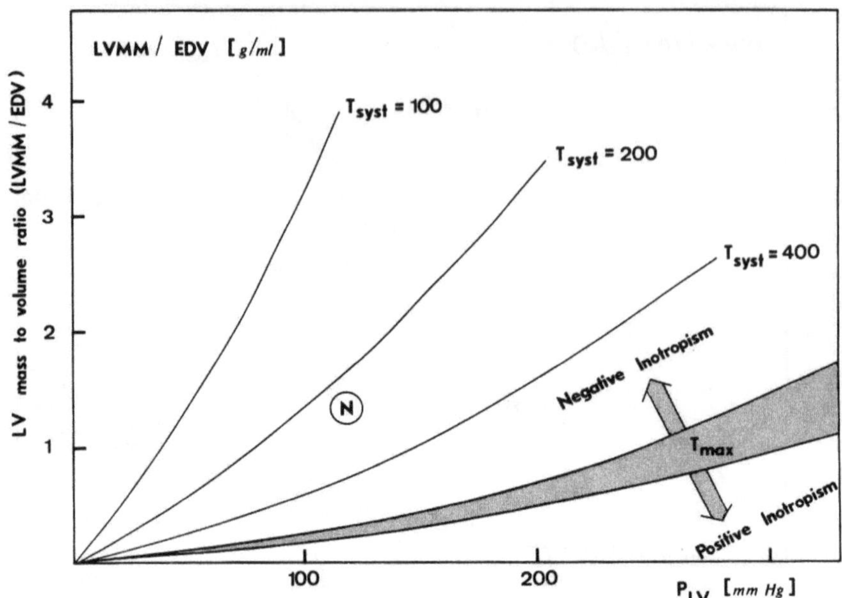

Fig. 51. Schematic diagram of the effects of negative or positive inotropic interventions on maximal achievable systolic wall stress (T_{max}). Changes in the wall stress and contractility reserve of the left ventricle are possible as a result of changes in T_{max}

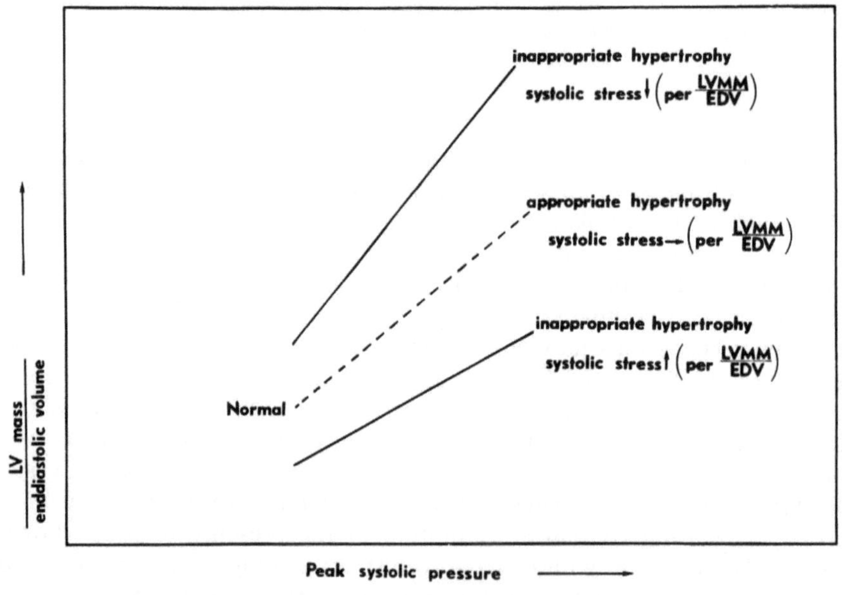

Fig. 52. Schematic diagram of the relationship between systolic pressure and mass-volume ratio with reference to the degree of proportionality of hypertrophy. The maximal systolic wall stress is lowered in overproportional hypertrophy, normal in proportional hypertrophy and increased in underproportional hypertrophy, i.e. in the presence of ventricular dilatation

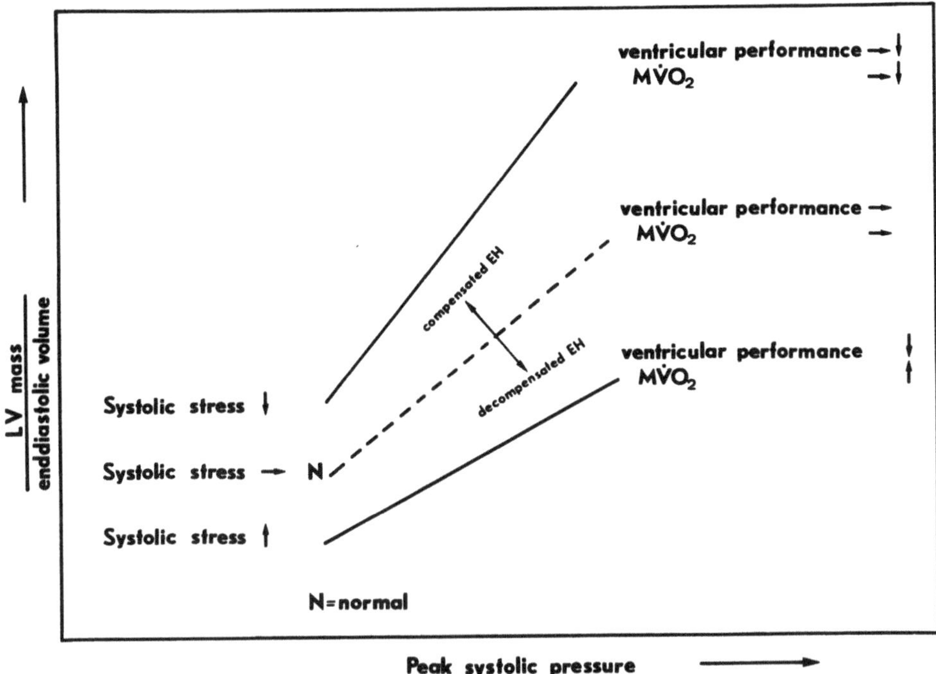

Fig. 53. Schematic diagram of the relationship between systolic pressure and mass-volume ratio. Note that there is an interrelation between systolic stress, ventricular function and oxygen consumption of the left ventricle

Apart from diagnostic or prognostic classification, the relationship between pressure, degree of hypertrophy and wall stress appear to be suitable for indicating the therapeutic value of drugs in the treatment of hypertensive heart disease (Figs. 54 and 55). In decompensated hypertensives a shift in the abnormal function curves is also achieved in the following two ways:

1. As a result of arterial pressure reduction, i.e. via non-negative inotropic antihypertensive drugs, pressure reduction and a decrease in wall stress can be expected.
2. Positive inotropic measures can produce an increase in the ejection fraction via long-term diminution of the heart size associated with a decrease in the end-diastolic volume. Moreover, the abnormal mass-volume ratio is increased by a reduction in the end-diastolic volume.

The concomitant use of both therapeutic measures, pressure reduction and positive inotropism, may have additive effects so that in compensated hypertensives the combined use of digitalis glycosides and antihypertensive drugs is indicated.

However, patients suffering from compensated and over-proportionally hypertrophied hypertension above all depend on the therapeutic measures which bring about a normalisation of the increased mass-volume ratio. Since ventricular function is normal or increased, no positive inotropic substances are indicated.

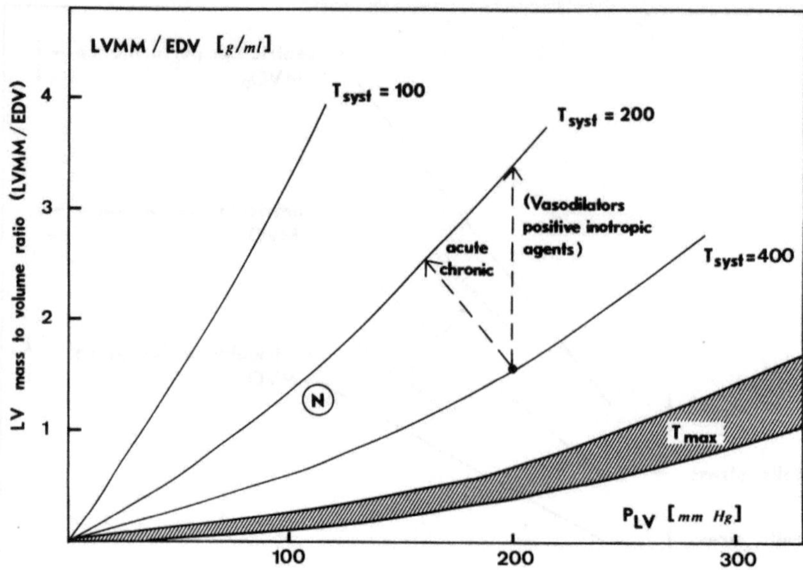

Fig. 54. Schematic diagram of the relationships between systolic pressure in the left ventricle (P_{LV}) and mass-volume ratio during treatment with positive inotropic drugs and vasodilators. Reduction in heart size, i.e. volume-relieving measures (acute: vasodilators; chronic: inotropic measures associated with diminution of the hearth size), lead to an increase in mass-volume ratio and hence a decrease in instantaneous systolic wall stress (T_{syst}). Thereby an increase in wall stress reserve, i.e. the quotient of peak wall stress (T_{max}) and instantaneous wall stress (T_{syst}), is possible

Regression of left ventricular muscle mass should be the prime concern and, as was seen from experiments with hypertensive and normotensive animals, it can achieved with varying success by chronic treatment with antihypertensive drugs (such as alpha-methyldopa, beta-receptor blocking agents) [114, 117]. The degree to which this reasonable concept (Sect. 3.8) will be of long-term therapeutic value in the treatment of essential hypertension in human beings, consisting in a change in mass-volume ratio, remains to be seen from follow-up studies in patients suffering from essential hypertension.

3.8 Ventricular Function and Myocardial Oxygen Consumption Under the Influence of Digitalis Glycosides (Digoxin)

This section deals with the findings on ventricular function, coronary haemo-dynamics (coronary blood flow), coronary vascular resistance, arteriocoronary venous oxygen difference and myocardial oxygen balance in 12 patients with essential hypertension with cardiac compensation under the acute influence of digitalis glycosides (digoxin).

The investigations involved diagnostic cardiac catheterisations and coronary angiographies (Table 13). All catheters were introduced using the Seldinger method. Apart from the local anaesthetic (xylocaine) there was no pre-medication.

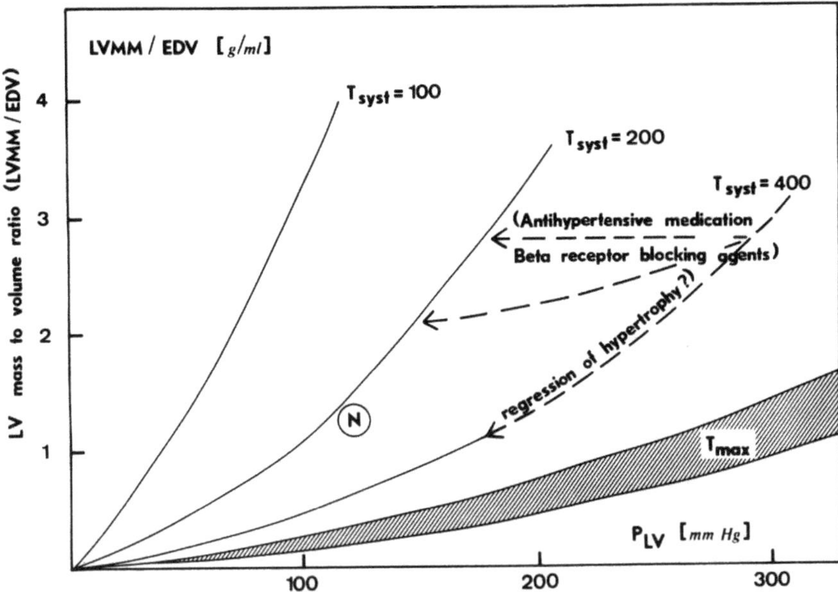

Fig. 55. Schematic diagram of the relationships between systolic pressure in the left ventricle (P_{LV}) and mass-volume ratio during acute and chronic pressure reduction. Acute pressure reduction, e. g. with antihypertensive measures, leads to a decrease in systolic pressure and thus to a proportional decrease in peak systolic wall stress. This allows a shifting to another isostress range associated with a corresponding increase in wall stress reserve and contractility reserve of the left ventricle. In contrast, in chronic pressure reduction with consecutive regression of ventricular wall hypertrophy (mass) and decrease in end-diastolic volume both a downward shifting within the same isostress range or a shift to another isostress range may occur. Accordingly, in the presence of arterial hypertension an increase in wall stress reserve and contractility reserve of the left ventricle can be achieved by means of both acute pressure reduction and chronic pressure relief

After local anaesthesia and introduction of the required catheters (left ventricle or aorta, coronary sinus and right atrium), digoxin (Lanicor, 0.01 mg/kg body weight) was slowly administered intravenously over a 5-min period. 10 and 5 min before as well as 15, 30 and 50 min after the digitalis injection, heart rate, left ventricular pressure, aortic blood pressure, cardiac output (thermodilution method) and derived parameters were measured, i. e. determined. The arteriocoronary venous oxygen saturation (CO-oximetry) was measured simultaneously. Left ventricular coronary blood flow was determined by means of the argon method 5 min before and 50 min after the intravenous digoxin injection.

Results

Case Material. The 12 patients (8 men, 4 women; mean age, 40 years) showed cardiac compensation according to the criteria of the New York Heart Association. In nine the case history was that of occasional attacks of angina pectoris and five

Table 13. Case material (digoxin study)

Number	n = 12
Age (years)	40
Degree of severity (122)	II
Duration of hypertension (years)	> 4
Angina pectoris	n = 9 (75%)
Dyspnoea at rest	–
Dyspnoea at exercise	n = 5 (42%)
Myocardial infarction	–
Cerebral haemorrhage	–
Left ventricular hypertrophy (chest X-ray)	n = 8 (67%)
(ECG)	n = 11 (92%)
Left atrial hypertrophy (ECG)	n = 9 (75%)
Coronary stenoses	–
Regional wall contraction disturbances	–
Coronary reserve (R_{cor}/R_{cor}*)	3.1
Irregular ventricular hypertrophy	n = 2 (17%)
Left ventricular muscle mass	194 g/m^2
End-diastolic volume	86 ml/m^2
Mass–volume ratio	1.73

* 0.5 mg/kg dipyridamole i.v.

possibly showed slight exertional dyspnoea. Eleven patients exhibited electrocardiographic signs of left ventricular hypertrophy, while in eight the chest X-ray showed left ventricular hypertrophy. With regard to case history, none of the patients exhibited symptoms of a previous myocardial infarction. The mean muscular mass of the left ventricle, which was determined by ventriculography, was 194 g/cm^2 and was thus 80% above our normal value (Table 13). With a mean of 86 ml/m^2 the end-diastolic volume was within the normal range, so that a considerable left ventricular hypertrophy with an increase in the mass-volume ratio to 1.73 was present. A coronary artery disease of the large coronary arteries could be excluded in all patients by selective coronary angiography. However, in eight patients the coronary reserve of the left ventricle (quotient of coronary vascular resistances before and after administration of 0.5 mg/kg dipyridamole i.v.) was 3.1 – a clear reduction. There were no regional wall contraction disturbances of the left ventricle (hypo-, a-, and dyskinesis). However, two patients exhibited an irregular or asymmetric anterior wall hypertrophy without signs of a ventriculo-arterial pressure gradient or intraventricular obstruction.

Ventricular Function (Table 14, Figs. 56, 57). Before treatment with digoxin the ventricular function, which can be determined by means of the cardiac index, the stroke index and the ejection fraction of the left ventricle (mean, 74%), was normal. With 2250 mm Hg/s the maximum rate of left ventricular pressure generation already showed a pressure-dependent increase before the digoxin injection. Fifty minutes after the digoxin injection it was possible to demonstrate a marked increase in the maximum rate of pressure generation (by 19.4%) independent of pressure and

74

Table 14. Mean values, standard deviations, significance (*t*-test for paired differences) and percentage changes before and 50 min after intravenous injection of digoxin (0,01 mg/kg) in 12 patients with essential hypertension with cardiac compensation. P_{LV}, systolic pressure in the left ventricle; P_{LVED}, end-diastolic pressure in the left ventricle; dp/dt_{max}, maximum rate of pressure generation in the left ventricle; TTI, approximation formula of the tension time index resulting from the product mean systolic pressure and the heart rate; V_{cor}, coronary blood flow of the left ventricle; R_{cor}, coronary vascular resistance; avDO, arteriocoronary venous oxygen difference; $M\dot{V}O_2$, myocardial oxygen consumption; n. s., not significant

	Digoxin			
	Before	After	P	%
P_{LV} (mm Hg)	196 ± 23	198 ± 21	n. s.	+ 1.1
P_{LVED} (mm HG)	15.9 ± 3.8	15.7 ± 3.1	n. s.	− 1.2
dp/dt_{max}	2 250 ± 287	2 687 ± 243	$P < 0.001$	+ 19.4
Heart rate (l/min)	74 ± 13	71 ± 12	n. s.	− 5.2
Cardiac index (liter/min · m²)	3.67 ± 0.57	3.26 ± 0.58	$P < 0.001$	− 11.2
Stroke index (ml/stroke · m²)	50.9 ± 12.5	47.6 ± 12	n. s.	− 6.5
Cardiac work (mm Hg · ml/min ·m²)	675 ± 86	610 ± 91	$P < 0.005$	− 9.7
$\sim$TTI ($\sim P_{syst} \cdot$ n)	13 828 ± 2 927	13 296 ± 2 652	n. s.	− 3.8
V_{cor} (ml/min · 100 g)	74.4 ± 14.2	67.8 ± 13.1	$P < 0.01$	− 8.8
R_{cor} (mm Hg · min · 100 g · ml⁻¹)	1.54 ± 0.21	1.71 ± 0.19	$P < 0.001$	+ 11
avDO₂ (Vol%)	12.15 ± 1.29	12.95 ± 1.17	$P < 0.001$	+ 5.9
MVO₂ (ml/min · 100 g)	9.03 ± 2.14	8.82 ± 1.83	n. s.	− 2.1

$\bar{x} \pm SD$, n = 12

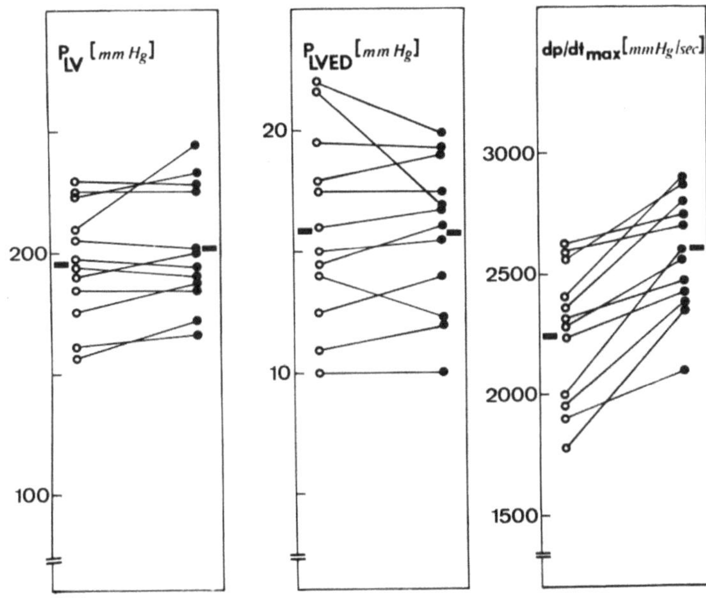

Fig. 56. Systolic pressure in the left ventricle (P_{LV}), end-diastolic pressure in the left ventricle (P_{LVED}) and maximum rate of pressure generation in the left ventricle (dp/dt_{max}) before and after administration of digoxin. As in subsequent figures, the black bars on the left and right margins show the mean values before and after administration of the agent. ○ before ● 50 min after digoxin 0.01 mg/kg i. v.

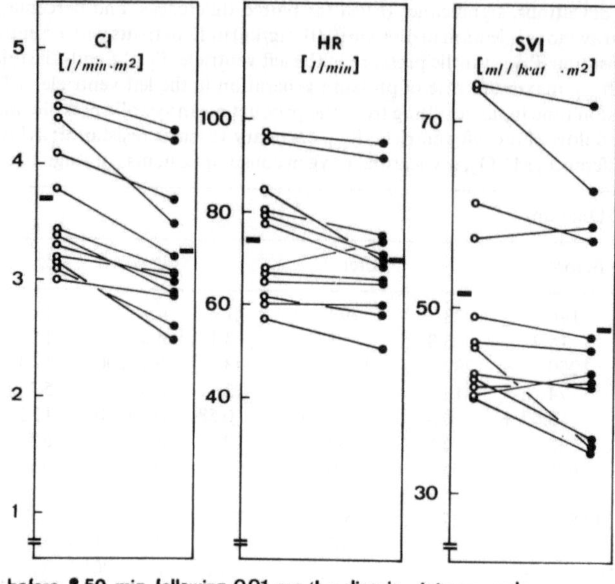

Fig. 57. Cardiac index (CI), heart rate (HR) and stroke volume index (SI) before and after administration of digoxin. ○ before ● 50 min after digoxin 0.01 mg/kg i.v.

heart rate, a fall in the cardiac index (by 11.2%) and − resulting from the changes in the mean systolic pressure and cardiac index − a reduction in the external cardiac work by 9.7%). Heart rate and stroke index were reduced by 5.2 and 0.5% respectively, which was without statistical significance. Left ventricular end-diastolic pressure remained practically unchanged. Corresponding to the arterial pressure elevation and the reduction in the cardiac index, total peripheral resistance was significantly increased (by 14.9%).

Coronary Haemodynamics and Myocardial Oxygen Consumption (Table 14, Fig. 58). Before treatment with digoxin, coronary blood flow and myocardial oxygen consumption per 100 g left ventricular weight were slightly increased as compared to normal. The arteriocoronary venous oxygen difference was normal. The coronary vascular resistance was markedly increased due to arterial hypertension associated with an elevation of coronary perfusion pressure. Fifty minutes after the digoxin injection the coronary blood flow was significantly reduced (by 8.8%) whereas the coronary vascular resistance and arteriocoronary venous oxygen difference increased by 11% and 5.9% respectively. Left ventricular oxygen consumption remained largely unchanged, showing a slight fall of 2.1%.

Discussion of the Results

The investigations show that a considerable increase in inotropism and a slight decrease in the pumping values of the left ventricle represent the main effects of

76

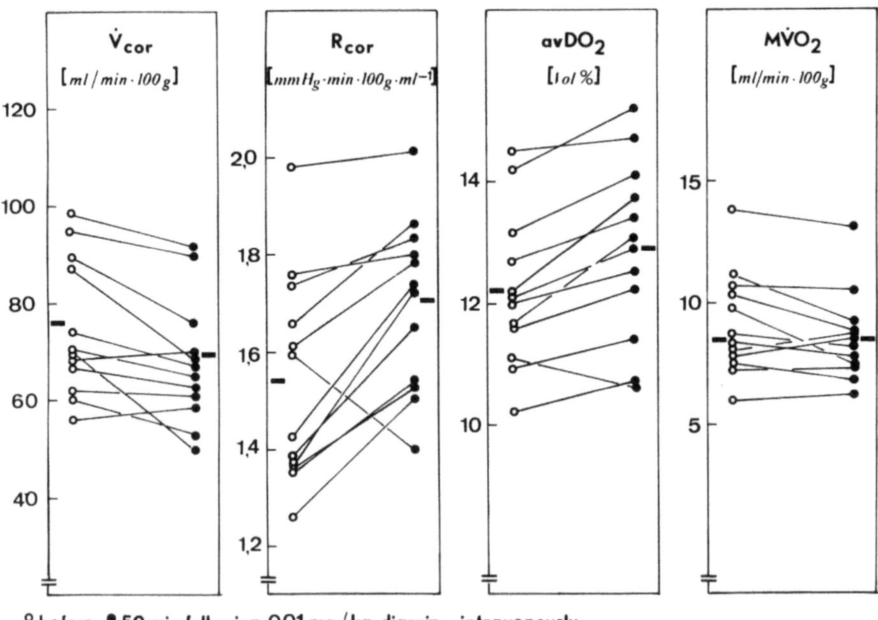

Fig. 58. Coronary blood flow (V_{cor}), coronary resistance (R_{cor}), arteriocoronary venous oxygen difference (avDO$_2$) and oxygen consumption of the left ventricle (MV̇O$_2$) before and after administration of digoxin. ○ before ● 50 min after digoxin 0.01 mg/kg i.v.

intravenously administered digoxin (0.01 mg/kg body weight) on the ventricular function in essential hypertension with cardiac compensation and a normal coronary angiogram. The changes in coronary haemodynamics were characterised by a marked decrease in coronary blood flow and an increase in coronary vascular resistance and arteriocoronary venous oxygen difference, while the myocardial oxygen consumption remained largely unchanged. As a result there was an increase in oxygen extraction associated with a decrease in coronary blood flow. Thus a haemodynamic situation was present, just as it sometimes occurs under coronary constrictive influence [7, 8, 17–19, 32, 105].

The increase in the maximum rate of left ventricular pressure generation associated with largely unchanged end-diastolic and systolic pressure shows that digoxin has a positive inotropic action on the hypertensive heart with cardiac compensation. This finding is in line with the digitalis-induced inotropic changes in the normotensive left ventricle (90). However, this left ventricular inotropic increase was paralleled by a fall in the parameters of the pumping function (cardiac index, stroke index, cardiac work). This is partly frequency-related but can also be explained by the co-existent increase in left ventricular impedance [14, 15, 66], which can be assessed on the basis of the changed total peripheral resistance having increased by 14.9%.' The result is that i.v. administration of digoxin causes a further increase in the peripheral resistance, which is anyway increased in essential hypertension, and that this increase can suffice to cause a decrease in left ventricular pumping function despite increased inotropism. This implies further that the considerable positive inotropic action of digoxin on the hypertensive heart with cardiac compensation is rather a luxus inotropism and is not suited to compensate for an afterload-dependent decrease of the pumping function. As left ventricular end-diastolic pressure remains largely unchanged, the fall in the stroke index and the external cardiac work, i. e. the stroke work of the left ventricle, imply that under digoxin the left ventricular function curve i. e. the relationship between end-diastolic pressure and cardiac work has been shifted downwards to lower ejection volumes. In the insufficient heart such a reduction in ventricular function can be improved or normalised by drugs with a positive inotropic action. [93]. In the compensated hypertensive heart an opposite effect has to be expected on the basis of present findings. This means that digoxin, despite a considerable positive inotropic action, does not improve ventricular function in essential hypertension with cardiac compensation, i.e. that in essential hypertension with cardiac compensation — contrary to decompensated essential hypertension — digoxin cannot transform the considerable increase in inotropism into an improved ventricular pumping function which is effective and therapeutically useful.

Corresponding to the ventriculodynamic determinants of myocardial energy demand, an increased oxygen consumption of the left ventricle would have to be expected as a result of the digoxin-induced inotropic increase [17, 19, 93]. The findings show that after administration of digoxin the myocardial oxygen consumption remaind practically unchanged despite a significant increase in inotropism. Accordingly it can be assumed that the change in the maximum rate of left ventricular pressure generation does not exert an equally pronounced influence on myocardial oxygen consumption or that the balance of other parameters of oxygen consumption has been reduced.

This primarily concerns the reductions in heart rate, cardiac index, stroke index and external cardiac work. There is little probability of a balance change of the systolic and/or diastolic wall stress as a result of digoxin because systolic and end-diastolic pressure in the left ventricle remained practically constant.

Corresponding to the reduced coronary blood flow, the increased coronary vascular resistance and the increased arteriocoronary venous oxygen difference, a slight coronary constrictive effect has to be expected after administration of digoxin in essential hypertension with cardiac compensation. As there is no simultaneous metabolic relief of the left ventricle, the high and unchanged myocardial oxygen consumption is compensated for by an increased oxygen extraction of left ventricular coronary blood flow. The potential causes include receptor effect and a direct effect on vascular smooth muscle (7, 17–19, 118). It is conceivable that in essential hypertension the increased coronary vascular resistance and the decreased coronary blood flow may cause a deterioration in the oxygen supply of the myocardium, which is already more sensitive to ischaemia due to left ventricular hypertrophy. In this context stenosis of the large coronary arteries need not be present because — as has been shown in our studies — the hypertensive heart with no pathological findings revealed by coronary angiography, of normal size and with cardiac compensation can already show a marked impairment of the coronary reserve and thus of the coronary regulatory capacity. Irrespective of whether there is a coronary macro-angiopathy, a coronary micro-angiopathy [43] or a normal coronary arterial system with attendant ventricular hypertrophy associated with essential hypertension, digoxin would not only be unsuited for improving ventricular function in essential hypertension with cardiac compensation but moreover would have the potential to cause a deterioration in the myocardial oxygen supply as a result of the increased coronary vascular resistance and the decreased coronary blood flow. Accordingly, it cannot be concluded that digitalis glycosides are indicated in essential hypertension with cardiac compensation. It must, however, be noted that these conclusions are based on findings achieved on the basis of acute actions of digoxin in essential hypertension. It is conceivable that variations in the acute action profile may occur under the conditions of chronic digoxin administration.

3.9 Ventricular Function, Coronary Blood Flow, Coronary Reserve and Myocardial Oxygen Consumption Under the Influence of Beta-Blocking Agents (Atenolol)

It is the aim of this section to examine the effects of an acute beta-blockade induced by intravenous administration of atenolol on the ventricular function, coronary haemodynamics and myocardial oxygen consumption in patients with essential hypertension and cardiac compensation.

The investigations were carried out in 11 such patients (Table 15). Between 8 and 10 days before the beginning of the study every pre-medication was discontinued. All patients were hospitalised and most of them observed strict confinement to bed.

Table 15. Case material (atenolol study)

Number		11
Age (years)		37
Degree of severity (122)		11
Duration of hypertension (years)		>2
Angina pectoris		7 (63%)
Dyspnoea at rest		–
Exertional dyspnoea		2 (18%)
Myocardial infarction		1 (9%)
Cerebral haemorrhage		–
Left ventricular hypertrophy (chest X-ray)		11 (100%)
(ECG)		10 (91%)
Left atrial hypertrophy (ECG)		8 (72%)
Coronary stenoses		3 (27%)
Regional wall contraction disturbances		–
Coronary reserve $(R_{cor}/R_{cor})^a$	$n=8$	2.61
	$n=3$ (with CHD)	2.21
	$n=5$ (without CHD)	3.01
Irregular ventricular hypertrophy		1
Left ventricular muscle mass		148 g/m^2
End-diastolic volume		91 ml/m^2
Mass–volume ratio		1.64

[a] dipyridamole (0.5 mg/kg i.v.)

After local anaesthesia (1% Xylocaine), the required catheters (left ventricle or aorta, right atrium, coronary sinus) were introduced using the Seldinger method. Before measuring the control values twice, i.e. 10 and 5 min before the injection of the beta-blocker, a haemodynamic balance was awaited in each patient over a period of 30 min. As beta-receptor blocking agent 5 mg atenolol was slowly administered over 5 min. 10, 20 and 30 min after the injection, heart rate, left ventricular pressure, aortic blood pressure, cardiac output (thermodilution method) and derived parameters were measured, i.e. determined. Five minutes before and 30 min after the intravenous atenolol injection, left ventricular coronary blood flow was determined by means of the argon method.

Results

Case Material. In seven patients the case history was one of angina pectoris (Table 15). Two patients exhibited slight exertional dyspnoea, and one had experienced a myocardial infarction. There were no signs of an antecedent cerebral haemorrhage. The roentgenograms of all patients showed signs of left ventricular hypertrophy; in ten patients there were electrocardiographic signs of left ventricular hypertrophy. In three patients the coronary angiogram revealed marked coronary stenoses. Two of these patients had high-grade stenoses (70%–90%) of the anterior descending left coronary artery and the diagonal branches of the left coronary artery, and one showed a co-existent 60% stenosis of the right coronary artery. The coronary angiograms of the other eight patients were normal. None of the treated patients showed regional wall contraction disturbances of the left ventricle. The coronary reserve of the left ventricle, which was determined by intravenous injection of 0.5 mg/kg dipyridamole in eight patients, including the three with coronary artery disease confirmed by coronary angiography, averaged 2,61 and was thus markedly impaired as compared to normal. In the three patients with coronary artery disease confirmed by coronary angiography, the coronary reserve was 2.21, while the coronary reserve of the hypertensives which no pathological findings in the coronary angiography was 3,01, i.e. it was also impaired. One patient exhibited ventriculographic signs of irregular ventricular wall hypertrophy but without intraventricular obstruction. The mean left ventricular muscle mass was 148 g/m², the end-diastolic volume, 91 ml/m². From this resulted a left ventricular mass-volume ratio which, at 1.64, was markedly increased as compared to normal.

Ventricular Function. During the measuring period (30 min) systolic pressure fell by 5.4% (Table 16, Fig. 59). There was no change in left ventricular end-diastolic pressure. The maximum rate of pressure generation was significantly reduced by 7.5%. There was a pronounced reduction (13.8%) in the heart rate. As the stroke index practically remained unchanged the reduced cardiac index has to be regarded as frequency dependent (Fig. 60). Cardiac work i.e. cardiac performance, and product of pressure and heart rate decreased by 14.3 and 19.2% respectively, corresponding to the changes in mean systolic pressure, cardiac index and heart rate.

Coronary Haemodynamics and Myocardial Oxygen Consumption. Left ventricular coronary blood flow showed a considerable reduction by 14.5% (Table 16, Fig. 61).

Table 16. Ventricular function and coronary haemodynamics before and 30 min after injection of 5 mg atenolol. P_{LV}, left ventricular systolic pressure; P_{LVED}, left ventricular end-diastolic pressure; dp/dt$_{max}$, maximum rate of pressure generation in the left ventricle; TTI, approximation formula of the tension-time index as product of pressure and heart rate from the mean systolic pressure and heart rate; V_{cor}, left ventricular coronary blood flow; R_{cor}, coronary vascular resistance; avDO$_2$, arteriocoronary venous oxygen difference; $M\dot{V}O_2$, left ventricular oxygen consumption; n.s., not significant

	Atenolol Before		After		P	%
P_{LV} (mm Hg)	189 ±	20	179 ±	17	<0.001	− 5.4
P_{LVED} (mm Hg)	15.4 ±	2.5	15 ±	14	n. s.	− 2.4
p/dt$_{max}$ (mm Hg)	2 260 ±	470	2 090 ±	359	<0.01	− 7.5
Heart rate (liter/min)	80 ±	9	69 ±	9	<0.001	− 13.8
Cardiac index (liter/min)	3.43 ±	0.45	3.03 ±	0.32	<0.001	− 11.5
Stroke index (ml/stroke · m²)	43.3 ±	4.12	43.8 ±	5.31	n. s.	+ 1.2
Cardiac work (mm Hg · ml/min · m²)	612 ±	84	524 ±	61	<0.001	− 14.3
∼TTI (P$_{syst}$ · n)	14 481 ±	2 539	11 713 ±	1 699	<0.001	− 19.2
V_{cor} (ml/min · 100 g)	86.4 ±	9.8	73,9 ±	12.5	<0.005	− 14.5
R_{cor} (mm Hg · min · 100 g · ml^{-1})	1.57 ±	0.32	1.76 ±	0.32	<0.005	+ 12.7
avDO$_2$ (vol. %)	12.26 ±	1.01	12.20 ±	0.95	n. s.	− 0.44
$M\dot{V}O_2$ (ml/min · 100 g)	10.43 ±	1.23	9.01 ±	1.40	<0.005	− 13.6

x̄ ± SD, n = 11

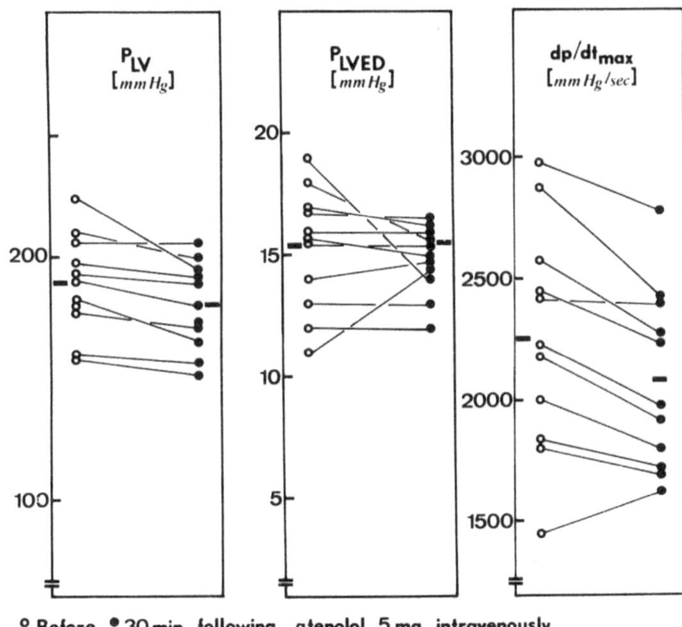

Fig. 59. Systolic pressure in the left ventricle (P_{LV}), end-diastolic pressure in the left ventricle (P_{LVED}) and maximum rate of pressure generation (dp/dt$_{max}$) before and after administration of atenolol. ○ before ● 30 min after atenolol 5 mg i.v.

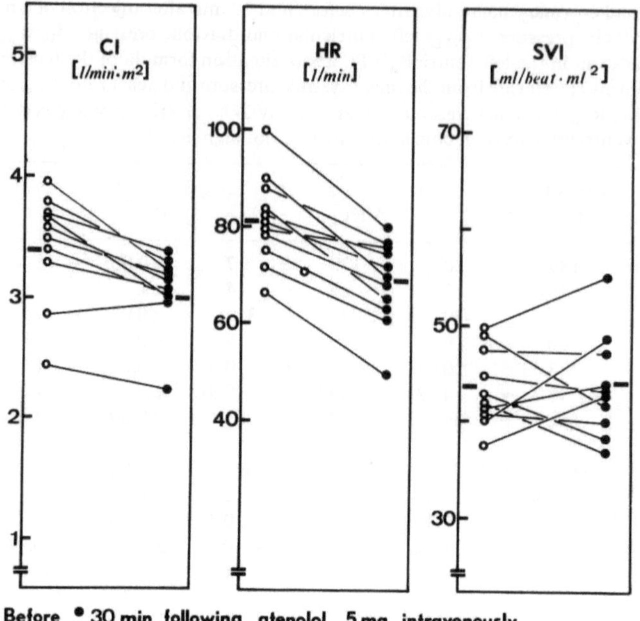

Fig. 60. Cardiac index (CI) heart rate (HR) and stroke volume index (SVI) before and after administration of atenolol. ○ before ● 30 min after atenolol 5 mg i.v.

The coronary vascular resistance increased markedly (12.7%), while the coronary perfusion pressure (mean diastolic aortic blood pressure less mean diastolic pressure of left ventricle) showed only a slight change. A definite alteration in arteriocoronary venous oxygen difference could not be demonstrated. Left ventricular oxygen consumption was significantly reduced by 13.6%.

Discussion of the Results

The studies show that under acute beta blockade induced by atenolol (5 mg i.v.) there are frequency-dependent reductions in left ventricular function (cardiac index, cardiac work, dp/dt_{max}) in patients with essential hypertension with cardiac compensation. The slight reduction in systolic pressure could in addition contribute to the change in the maximum rate of pressure generation. Signs of a directly negative inotropic action of atenolol were not observed. The reductions in heart rate, cardiac index, dp/dt_{max}, cardiac work and tension-time index thus show an effective systolic relief of the left ventricle. The haemodynamic alterations were characterised by a marked decrease in coronary blood flow and myocardial oxygen consumption while the arteriocoronary venous oxygen difference remained unchanged. The coronary resistance increased considerably. Left ventricular systolic relief was thus associated with a marked metabolic relief, i.e. a reduction in myocardial energy demand (Fig. 62).

82

Atenolol can be classified as beta blocker with mainly cardioselective properties producing a pronounced fall in arterial pressure in arterial hypertension when chronically administered [1, 34, 72]. Apart from its antihypertensive effect its most pronounced effect is the reduction of the heart rate which becomes manifest under chronic application and is already seen as an acute effect and which is causally related to the fall in cardiac index, cardiac work, tension-time index and maximum rate of pressure generation. After acute intravenous administration of 5 mg atenolol the heart rate is reduced by 13.8% (Table 16), while after chronic oral application of 75–100 mg atenolol it is reduced by ca. 15%–18% (1) so that under these conditions the effects on the heart rates are quantitatively comparable. However, there is a marked difference in the effect on blood pressure after acute (-5.4%) and chronic application. Accordingly, after chronic application a stronger fall in cardiac performance and tension-time index has to be expected, followed by a still more pronounced fall in those parameters determining left ventricular oxygen consumption so that the fall in pressure and heart rate caused by atenolol has to be regarded as an effective correlate of left ventricular systolic relief: However, as far as the practical-therapeutic use of atenolol in essential hypertension is concerned, it has to be noted that, as a result of the pronounced fall in the heart rate, haemodynamic side-effects such as bradycardia-related high pressure peaks cannot be excluded.

In connection with the decrease in coronary blood flow and the increase in coronary vascular resistance under acute beta-blockade, among other things the

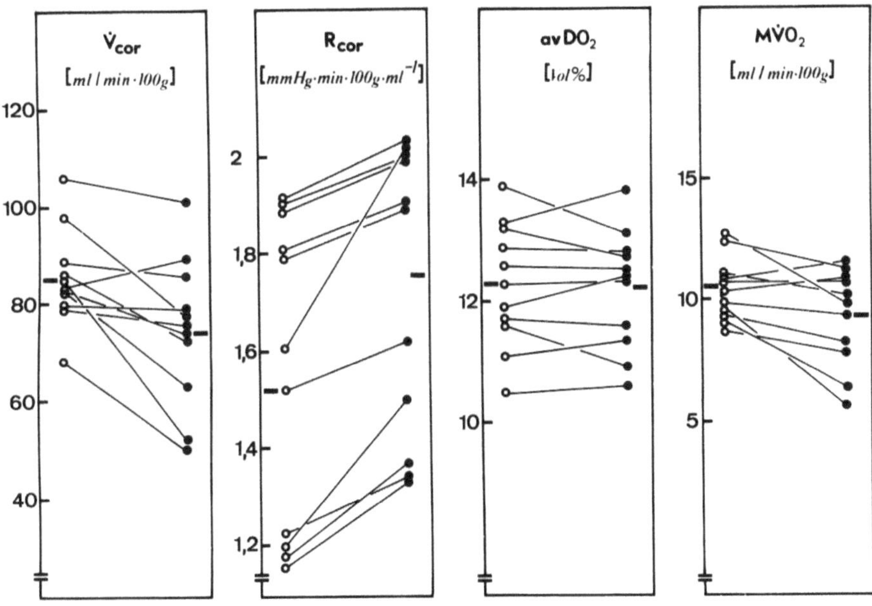

Fig. 61. Coronary blood flow of the left ventricle (V_{cor}), coronary resistance (R_{cor}), arteriocoronary venous oxygen difference (avDO₂) and myocardial oxygen consumption (MV̇O₂) before and after administration of atenolol. ○ before ● 30 min after atenolol 5 mg i.v.

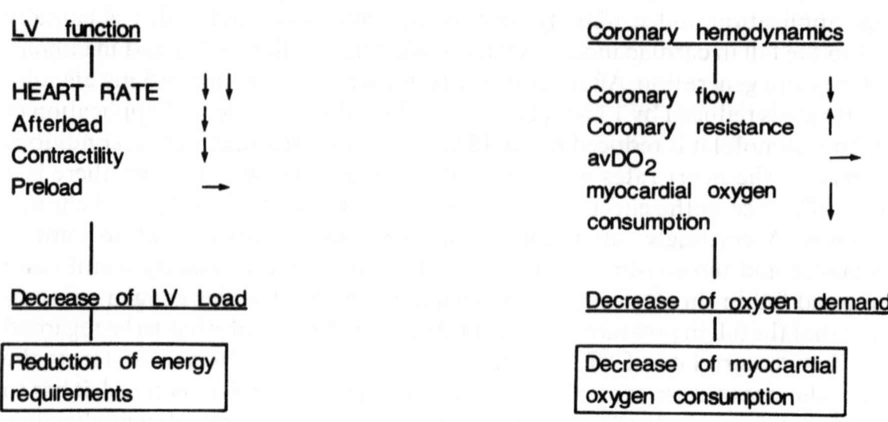

Fig. 62. Schematic representation of the haemodynamic effects of beta-receptor blockade

ventriculodynamic and metabolic effects of atenolol, the changes in the activities of beta-receptors and the direct effect on vascular smooth muscle of the coronary arterial system have to be discussed [60, 69, 70, 74, 76, 118]. Assuming that alpha- and beta-receptors do exist in the coronary vascular system in man, a beta-blockade could lead to a relative dominance of alpha-receptors followed by coronary constriction (increase in coronary vascular resistance, decrease in coronary blood flow). However, given this haemodynamic condition an increase in coronary oxygen extraction, which is measurable by the increase in the arteriocoronary venous oxygen difference, would have to be expected. As the arteriocoronary venous oxygen difference remained unchanged a primary coronary constriction caused by the dominance of alpha-receptors or by a possible direct effect of atenolol on coronary constriction can largely be excluded. What is more probable is that the fall in myocardial oxygen consumption is due to the decrease of its ventriculodynamic determinants in the presence of high coronary oxygen extraction and that the decrease in myocardial energy demand after administration of atenolol is followed by a reduction in coronary blood flow and an increase in coronary vascular resistance. In this respect the changes in coronary blood flow and coronary vascular resistance have to be regarded as metabolic changes and primarily as the result of the changed myocardial energy demand under beta-blockade. In five patients with essential hypertension with cardiac compensation the coronary reserve was determined under control conditions as well as after intravenous administration of 0.5 mg dipyridamole per kilogram body weight 40 min after intravenous injection of 5 mg atenolol and was found to have risen by 21% (Table 17). The minimum coronary vascular resistance which could be achieved was practically the same with and without atenolol, whereas the initial value was markedly higher after atenolol. This means that the increase in the coronary reserve has to be regarded as a result of

Table 17. Coronary blood flow (V_{cor}), coronary vascular resistance (R_{cor}) before and after dipyridamole and left ventricular coronary reserve under control conditions and after beta-blockade using 5 mg atenolol i.v. Note the increase in the coronary reserve after atenolol.

V_{cor} (ml/min · 100)	R_{cor} (mm Hg · min ·	R_{cor}^{a} 100 g · ml^{-1})	Coronary reserve ($R_{cor}/R_{cor}a$)
Control 89.2	1.61	0.53	3.03
Atenolol 74.8	1.79	0.49	3.66

[a] 0.5 mg/kg dipyridamole i.v.

the increased coronary vascular resistance after administration of atenolol [97, 98]. This implies further that when causing a ventriculodynamic and metabolic relief an increased coronary regulatory capacity has to be expected despite a resultant increase in coronary vascular resistance and decrease in coronary blood flow. Probably this increase in the coronary reserve finds its clinical correlate in an improved exercise tolerance and a reduced pain sensitivity in coronary patients with or without arterial hypertension who have been treated with beta-blockers. Recently our study group has reported similar findings in coronary artery disease without arterial hypertension [97, 98]. It is conceivable that other interventions such as negative inotropic, negative chronotropic and antihypertensive drugs causing metabolic relief associated with a decrease in coronary blood flow and myocardial oxygen consumption and an increase in coronary vascular resistance can produce an increase in the coronary reserve and thus in coronary tolerance. In this respect an improvement in the coronary reserve of the heart can be expected due to the reduction of the mechanical and haemodynamic determinants of myocardial energy demand achieved by negative inotropic and negative chronotropic measures, whereas conversely, interventions leading to an increased myocardial oxygen consumption are usually accompanied by a decrease in coronary reserve.

The fall in the pumping function and the myocardial oxygen consumption under the influence of beta-blocking agents could possibly produce a regression of the abnormally increased left ventricular muscle mass in essential hypertension with concentric or irregular hypertrophy and cardiac compensation by long-term reduction of heart rate, velocity of contraction and cardiac performance. In this way the increased mass-volume ratio could be decreased. Animal experiments have shown that it is possible to reduce ventricular hypertrophy in normotensive as well as in hypertensive animals by means of long-term beta-blockade. Follow-up studies in patients with essential hypertension will show to what extent this sensible concept — after the appropriate change in the mass-volume ratio has been made — is of long-term therapeutic value for the treatment of essential hypertension in man.

3.10 Ventricular Function, Coronary Blood Flow and Myocardial Oxygen Consumption Under the Influence of Hydralazine

Vasodilating agents are increasingly being used in the failing heart in order to improve ventricular function by unloading of both preload and afterload. In hypertensive heart disease, reduction of the elevated arterial blood pressure is commonly associated with a corresponding reduction in systolic wall stress which represents the main determinant of left ventricular afterload. As has been demonstrated earlier in this monograph (see Fig. 40), an increase in systolic wall stress decreases left ventricular function, whereas stress reduction may improve cardiac performance. Therapeutic antihypertensive treatment runs parallel with cardiac unloading, and in some conditions, such as arterial and arteriolar vasodilatation, with an enhancement of cardiac performance. One of the most effective vasodilating antihypertensives is hydralazine. This study was therefore performed in order to analyse the effects of hydralazine on left ventricular function, on coronary haemodynamics and on myocardial oxygen consumption in patients with hypertensive heart disease.

Studies were carried out in ten patients with essential hypertension during diagnostic cardiac catheterisation. The methodological procedure has been described extensively in Chap. 2. The haemodynamic measurements were performed before (double measurements of control values at 5-min intervals, following a haemodynamic steady state of 30 min) and 30 min following the intravenous infusion (over 10 min) of 20 mg hydralazine. Coronary blood flow was determined by the argon method 5 min before and 30 min after hydralazine infusion.

Results

Case Material. All patients had essential hypertension for more than 4 years. The WHO severity degree was II/III; cardiac severity degree was, according to the NYHA classification, II (six cases), III (three cases) and IV (one case).

Eight patients had exertional angina pectoris; four had dyspnoea at rest and five at exercise. In two patients previous myocardial infarction was found. None of the patients had a history of cerebrovascular insult.

All patients had marked left ventricular hypertrophy, as evidenced by chest X-rays and by the ECG. Left atrial hypertrophy was found in five patients. Significant coronary artery stenoses were present in eight patients; in six regional wall contraction abnormalities could be detected by left ventriculography.

Coronary reserve averaged 2.91. One patient had irregular left ventricular hypertrophy. Left ventricular mass was markedly increased in all patients (Table 18), and there was left ventricular dilatation as revealed by the left ventriculogram (Table 18).

Ventricular Function. Under the influence of hydralazine (20 mg i. v.), left ventricular systolic pressure decreased by 16% (from 167 to 140 mm Hg), and left ventricular end-diastolic pressure markedly decreased by 27% (Table 19). There were no significant changes in heart rate nor in the maximum rate of left ventricular pressure development (dp/dt_{max}). Cardiac index and stroke volume index were enhanced by 24% and 18% respectively, whereas external cardiac work remained nearly unaltered as a consequence of reduction in systolic blood pressure and increase in cardiac output. The product of mean systolic pressure and heart rate significantly decreased by 15%, thus indicating effective ventricular unloading (Figs. 63, 64).

Table 18. Case material (hydralazine study)

Number	10
Age [years]	54
Severity degree [WHO report]	II/III
Severity degree [NYHA]	II (n = 6)
	III (n = 3)
	IV (n = 1)
EH duration [years]	4
Angina pectoris	8 (80%)
Dyspnoea at rest	4 (40%)
Dyspnoea at exercise	5 (50%)
Previous myocardial infarction	2 (20%)
Previous cerebrovascular insult	–
Left heart hypertrophy (chest x-ray	6 (60%)
ECG	10 (100%)
Left atrial hypertrophy	4 (40%)
Coronary artery stenosis	8 (80%)
Regional wall contraction abnormalities	1 (10%)
Irregular hypertrophy	1 (10%)
Left ventricular muscle mass (LVMM)	169 g/m^2
End-diastolic volume (EDV)	118 ml/m^2
LVMM/EDV	1.43

Coronary Haemodynamics. Coronary blood flow was considerably enhanced by 41% (from 59 to 83 ml/min · 100 g). The coronary vascular resistance decreased by 36% (from 1,71 to 1,09 units), and the arteriocoronary venous oxygen difference was markedly reduced. Myocardial oxygen consumption of the left ventricle was almost unchanged (Fig. 65).

Discussion

The results demonstrate that hydralazine leads to:

a) Effective ventricular unloading, as evidenced by reduction in both end-diastolic and systolic left ventricular pressure (Table 19).
b) Considerable augmentation of left ventricular ejection pump funtion.
c) Marked increase in coronary blood flow without significantly changing myocardial oxygen consumption.

One of the predominant effects of hydralazine is arterial and arteriolar dilatation. Thereby systolic left ventricular unloading may be achieved together with improvement in ejection pump parameters. Systolic unloading by hydralazine results from reduction in both left ventricular end-diastolic and systolic pressures:

a) Decrease in systolic pressure is associated with systolic stress reduction and thereby with lowering of the left ventricular afterload. In this case left ventricular geometry may remain unchanged.

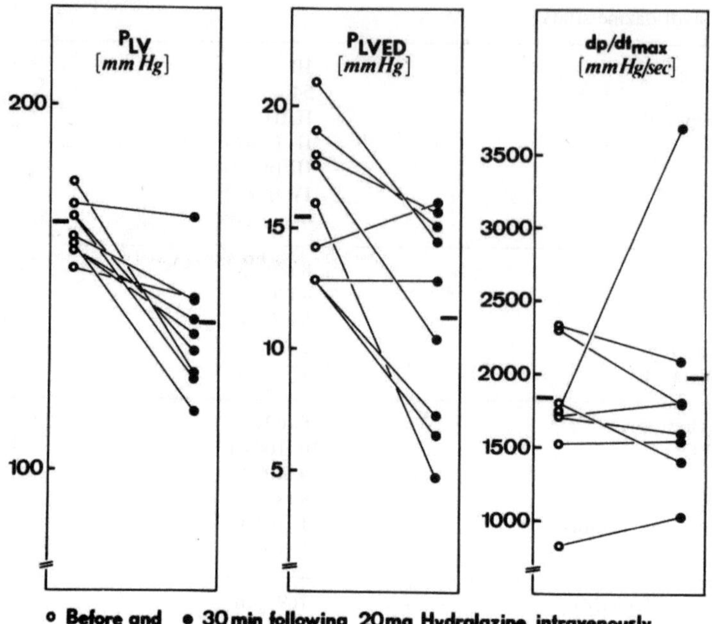

Fig. 63. Effects of hydralazine (20 mg i.v.) on systolic left ventricular pressure (P_{LV}), left ventricular end-diastolic pressure (P_{LVED}) and the maximum rate of left ventricular pressure development (dp/dt_{max})

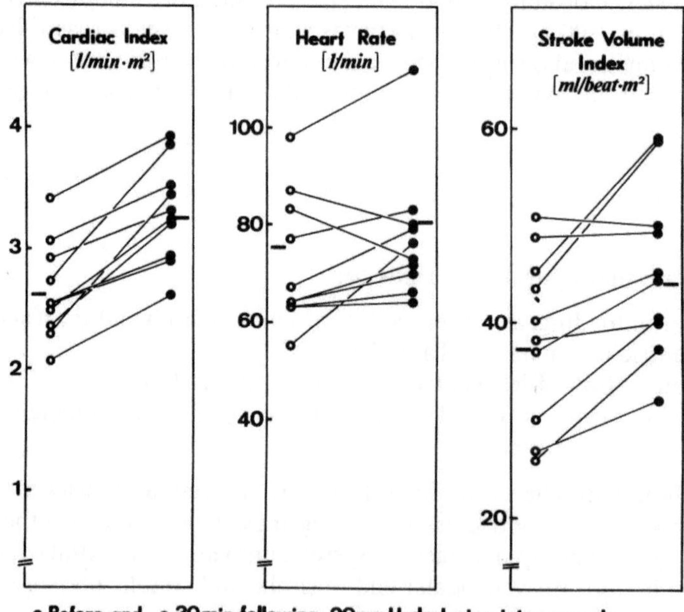

Fig. 64. Effects of hydralazine (20 mg i.v.) on cardiac index, heart rate and stroke volume index. Note the increases in cardiac pump parameters

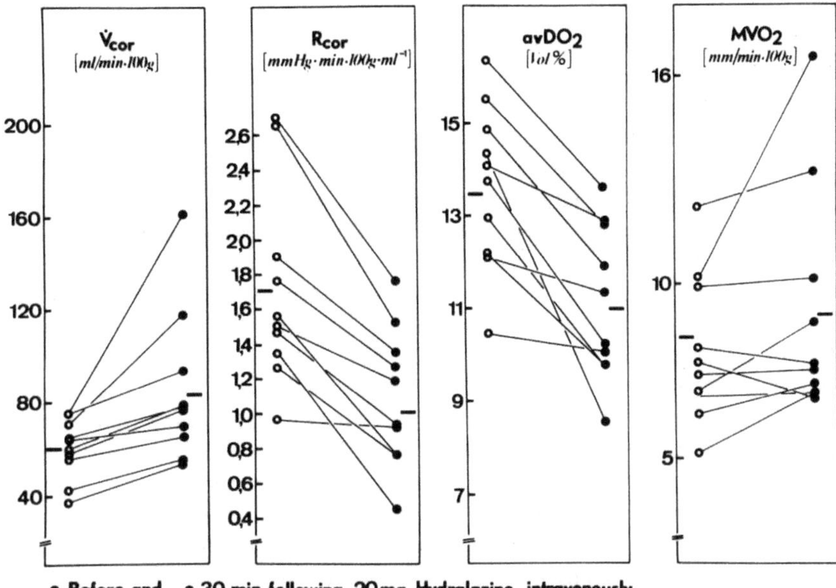

Fig. 65. Effects of hydralazine (20 mg i.v.) on coronary blood flow (V_{vor}), coronary vascular resistance (R_{cor}), arteriocoronary venous oxygen difference ($avDO_2$) and myocardial oxygen consumption ($M\dot{V}O_2$). Note the increase in coronary blood flow and decreased coronary resistance at nearly normal oxygen consumption

b) Decrease in end-diastolic pressure, even at constant systolic pressure, leads to diminution of left ventricular end-diastolic volume. The mass-volume ratio is then increased and systolic wall stress decreases.

Table 19. Acute hemodynamic effects of hydralazine on left ventricular function and coronary hemodynamics. Note the effective ventricular unloading as well as the coronary dilating capacity of hydralazine

	Hydralazine Before	After	P	%
P_{LV} [mm Hg]	167.2 ± 8.4	140.2 ± 16.4	<0.001	−16.12
P_{LVED} [mm Hg]	15.4 ± 3.4	11.2 ± 4.1	<0.01	−27.04
dp/dt_{max} [mm Hg/sec]	1836.3 ±513.5	1988.6 ±823.4	n.s.	+ 8.30
Heart rate [1/min]	75.0 ± 16.0	80.0 ± 16.0	n.s.	+ 6.8
Cardiac index [1/min · m²]	2.61± 0.38	3.25± 0.43	<0.001	+24.24
Stroke volume index [ml/beat · m²]	37.0 ± 9.7	43.8 ± 10.2	<0.005	+18.40
Cardiac work [mm Hg · ml/min · m²]	447.5 ± 58.7	480.6 ± 70.5	n.s.	+ 7.39
~TTI ($\bar{P}_{syst}$ · HR)	1088.1 ±243.6	920.1 ±138.6	<0.01	−15.44
$\dot{V}_{COR}$ [ml/min · 100 g]	59.4 ± 12.8	83.8 ± 33.0	<0.02	+41.13
R_{COR} [mm Hg · min · 100 g · ml⁻¹]	1.11± 0.57	1.09± 0.40	<0.01	−36.14
$avDO_2$ [Vol %]	13.47± 1.80	10.97± 1.63	<0.001	−18.58
$M\dot{V}O_2$ [ml/min · 100 g]	8.47± 2.34	9.10± 3.12	n.s.	+ 7.51

$\bar{x}$ ± SD, n = 10

As can be derived from the basic relationships between the mass-volume ratio and systolic wall stress (see Figs. 33, 40), reduction in systolic pressure usually leads to greater stress reduction than to a comparable reduction in end-diastolic pressure. On the other hand, reduction in systolic wall stress and hence in left ventricular afterload is still greater if both systolic pressure and end-diastolic pressure are reduced. This has been shown for hydralazine. Thus, one of the basic effects of hydralazine is effective left ventricular unloading.

The acute reduction in left ventricular afterload was accompanied by marked augmentation of ejection phase indexes. Since heart size decreased, an increased fibre shortening can be assumed, resulting in increased cardiac output and stroke volume index. This augmentation of auxotonic pump parameters of the left ventricle may be considered one of the most important target actions of hydralazine. It can be related, in the absence of direct inotropic effects, almost exclusively to the hydralazine-dependent changes in left ventricular geometry and afterload (and impedance) and hence in systolic wall stress. It is reasonable to assume that *chronic* application of hydralazine parallel with systolic pressure reduction may have a still greater effect on the improvement of left ventricular function.

External cardiac work remained nearly unchanged, since the decrease in pressure was nearly counterbalanced by the increases in cardiac output and stroke index. The tension-time index (pressure rate product) significantly decreased, since the pressure reduction was more pronounced than the fall in heart rate.

The coronary response to hydralazine were characterised by direct coronary vasodilatation. Coronary blood flow increased, coronary vascular resistance decreased and the arteriocoronary venous oxygen difference, which is equivalent to coronary oxygen extraction, fell significantly. This demonstrates luxus perfusion under the influence of hydralazine, and arteriolar dilatation therefore also seems to be present in the coronary vascular bed. There was no angina following hydralazine in these hypertensive patients.

The overall myocardial oxygen consumption remained normal. This means that the increase in myocardial oxygen consumption, as induced by the significant and non-significant increases in stroke volume index, external cardiac work, heart rate and dp/dt_{max} was counterbalanced by the oxygen-serving factors, primarily induced by systolic wall stress reduction. This again elucidates the importance of systolic wall stress for myocardial energy demand. Moreover, it demonstrates the beneficial mode of action of hydralazine, which considerably enhances left ventricular function without increasing myocardial oxygen consumption.

Thus, hydralazine can be considered a vasodilator with high therapeutic value in hypertensive heart disease, if preservation and/or improvement of ventricular function without alterations in myocardial energy demand are desired.

4 Summary

Between 1969 and 1980 *systematic studies* on *ventricular function, coronary haemodynamics* and *myocardial oxygen balance* were carried out for the first time in 158 patients with essential hypertension, included diagnostic cardiac catheterisations, coronary angiographies, ventriculographies and reno-angiographies. In addition, the determinants of the degree of left ventricular hypertrophy and oxygen consumption were analysed, and diagnostic possibilities and therapeutic consequences for the hypertensive heart were studied under control conditions and under the influence of digitalis glycosides, beta-blockers and hydralazine. The results can be summarised as follows:

1. In severe left ventricular hypertrophy, compensated essential hypertension without coronary artery disease is characterised by a normal or increased ventricular function at rest and during physical exercise. In the absence of regional wall contraction disturbances, compensated essential hypertension with coronary artery disease may show a normal ventricular function. When the end-diastolic volume increases and regional wall contraction anomalies occur, marked contraction disturbances of the whole left ventricle must be expected even at rest. According to cardially quantifiable criteria, decompensated essential hypertension is present if the left ventricle increases over-proportionally in relation to the degree of hypertrophy, so that with an increasing end-diastolic volume the ejection fraction decreases progressively.

2. The relationship between end-diastolic volume and ejection fraction is a characteristic feature of essential hypertension, by means of which it is possible to perform a functional assessment of left ventricular contraction. Left ventricular heart size, which can be identified by roentgenography, is of primary importance when classifying the clinical degree of essential hypertension and when evaluating therapeutic steps, because due to the inverse relationship between heart size and ejection fraction the determination of heart size represents a reliable parameter for the indirect determination of ventricular function.

3. With a largely normal arteriocoronary venous oxygen difference coronary perfusion pressure (+56%), coronary vascular resistance (+38%) and left ventricular coronary blood flow (+16%) are increased significantly as compared to normal. Left ventricular function in hypertensives with significant coronary stenoses is extremely impaired, as is the case in normotensive coronary artery disease with comparable coronary stenoses. However, a marked impairment of left ventricular coronary reserve can already be observed in patients with compensated essential hypertension and a normal coronary angiogram, a finding demonstrating

that coronary risk exists even for the hypertensive heart of normal size with a normal coronary angiogram.

4. Left ventricular oxygen consumption per weight unit shows a mean increase of 21% in the total group of hypertensives. There is a marked dependence on systolic well stress which is an essential determinant of myocardial oxygen consumption in essential hypertension. As systolic wall stress increases when ventricular dilatation increases, left ventricular size in essential hypertension not only represents a clinically useful correlate for determining ventricular function but also an index for assessing the risk of left ventricular ischaemia.

5. Essential hypertension is accompanied by assymmetric or irregular ventricular wall hypertrophy in 14% of cases. There was a markedly higher incidence of maximal end-diastolic and end-systolic increases in wall thickness of ventricular segments with irregular hypertrophy (133%) as compared to normal (58%). Ventriculographic pictures resembling those of hypertrophic obstructive cardiomyopathy could be demonstrated formally, but in none of these cases was there an intraventricular or outflow tract obstruction. In comparison with hypertensives with regular hypertrophy and as against normal, the systolic wall stress in the ventricular wall segments with irregular hypertrophy was markedly reduced. All patients showed cardiac compensation and most exhibited significant coronary stenoses. It must be assumed that essential hypertension is the most frequent form of an irregular or asymmetric ventricular wall hypertrophy.

6. In compensated essential hypertension without coronary artery disease ventricular compliance is normal even in the presence of severe ventricular hypertrophy, whereas in coronary secondary diseases and decompensated hypertension there is a pronounced fall in compliance. Thus left ventricular hypertrophy in essential hypertension does not, in itself, imply an alteration in ventricular compliance. Decreasing ventricular compliance is accompanied by a decrease in the forward pumping performance, whereas ventricular performance (product of wall stress generated during systole and stroke volume) increases. This disproportion between external and internal ventricular performance becomes greater with increasing ventricular dilatation and is most pronounced in decompensated essential hypertension. Thus, in comparison with all other groups of hypertensives decompensated essential hypertension shows the highest ventricular performance and the lowest forward pumping function.

7. Peak systolic wall stress is an important resultant of the degree of hypertrophy and determines ventricular function and myocardial energy demand. On the basis of the degree of hypertrophy, i.e. of its proportionality, it is possible to define three forms of left ventricular hypertrophy which are in principle different:

a) an over-proportional hypertrophy with a high mass-volume ratio and a reduced wall stress,
b) a proportional hypertrophy with normal wall stress and
c) an under-proportional hypertrophy with a normal or decreased mass-volume ratio and an increased wall stress.

On the basis of the degree of hypertrophy and the functional classification of the hypertensive heart, drug therapies are presented, such as beta-blockers in over-proportional hypertrophy and digitalis glycosides in under-proportional hypertrophy.

8. In essential hypertension with cardiac compensation the effect of intravenously administered digoxin (0.01 mg/kg body weight) is reflected by a marked, velocity-related inotropic increase of the left ventricle by 19.4%, whereas the pumping function parameters (cardiac index, cardiac work, stroke index) decrease by between 6.5% and 11.2%. Left ventricular coronary blood flow was reduced by 8.8%, whereas coronary vascular resistance and arteriocoronary venous oxygen difference increased by 11% and 5.9% respectively. The oxygen consumption remained largely unchanged (-2.1%).

The findings show that the inotropic increase caused by the intravenous administration of digoxin in essential hypertension with cardiac compensation cannot only not be transformed into an improved left ventricular pumping function of therapeutic use but that in addition a slight coronary constrictive effect and a potential of risk ischaemia has to be expected in the coronary vascular system. Therefore the use of digoxin in compensated essential hypertension should be recommended with reservation.

9. In compensated essential hypertension a beta-blockade with atenolol (5 mg i.v.) leads to a slight decrease in arterial blood pressure (-5.4%), an unchanged inotropism and marked reductions in heart rate (-13.8%), cardiac index (-11.5%) and cardiac work (-14.3%). The alterations in coronary haemodynamics were characterised by pronounced falls in coronary blood flow (-14.5%) and myocardial oxygen consumption (-13.6%), while the arteriovenous oxygen difference was normal. There was a considerable increase in coronary vascular resistance ($+12.7\%$). The left ventricular coronary reserve, which was determined in five patients after administration of atenolol. increased by ca. 16%.

10. In hypertensive heart disease with concentric and with developing excentric left ventricular hypertrophy, hydralazine produces marked improvement in left ventricular function, as evidenced by the increases in cardiac index ($+24\%$) and stroke volume index ($+18\%$). There is marked coronary vasodilatation with increase in coronary blood flow ($+41\%$), decrease in coronary vascular resistance (-36%) and decrease in arteriocoronary venous oxygen difference (-18%). The myocardial oxygen consumption was nearly unchanged ($+7.5\%$), thus indicating effective improvement in left ventricular function without a significant increase in myocardial energy demand. This beneficial action of hydralazine is due to the effective systolic unloading (wall stress reduction, decrease in ventricular impedance) which counterbalances the energy costs associated with increased fibre shortening (increases in cardiac index and stroke volume index).

The findings show that acute beta-blockade in essential hypertension results in an effective systolic unloading of the left ventricle associated with an equivalent reduction in myocardial energy demand. It is concluded that the changes in coronary vascular resistance and the increase in left ventricular coronary reserve have to be regarded as a metabolic affect of a beta-blockade.

The results of the tests show that in essential hypertension, which is the most frequent form of left ventricular pressure load, the heart exhibits a syndrome of findings concerning ventricular function, degree of hypertrophy, coronary haemodynamics and myocardial energy balance which is specific for the cardial severity concerned and which depends on the hypertension and the consequences of hypertrophy (myocardial factor) as well as on the coronary organic manifestations of essential hypertension (coronary factor). By means of these constellations of findings it is possible for the first time to perform a diagnostic classification of the hypertrophied heart at rest and during exercise. According to the clinical findings, hypertension can be divided into four stages with regard to ventricular function, hypertrophy, coronary haemodynamics and central circulatory function:

Stage I: Rare heart complaints.
Normal heart silhouette, ventricular function and coronary angiogram
Possible irregular ventricular wall hypertrophy
Impairment of coronary reserve (+)

Stage II Frequent heart complaints in the presence of coronary heart disease (angina pectoris)
Heart silhouette and ventricular function (rest, exercise) still normal
Frequent irregular ventricular wall hypertrophy
Impairment of coronary reserve (+ + +)

Stage III Frequent complaints (angina pectoris, exertional dyspnoea)
Heart silhouette enlarged
Impaired of ventricular function and contractility during physical stress
Occasional irregular ventricular wall hyoertrophy

Stage IV Clinical signs of decompensated heart failure
Heart silhouette markedly enlarged
Impairment of ventricular function at rest
No irregular ventricular wall hypertrophy

By studying the function and mechanism of the hypertensive heart it has become possible to develop a clinically useful basis for classifying the different degrees of essential hypertension and for establishing a rational differential diagnosis.

5 References

1. Amery, H., Billiet, L., Boel, A., Fagard, R., Reybrouck, T., Willems, J.: Mechanism of hypotensive effect during beta-adrenergic blockade in hypertensive patients. Amer. Heart J. *91*, 634 (1976)
2. Bachmann, K., Zerzawy, R., Riess, P. J., Zölch, K. A.: Blutdrucktelemetrie – kontinuierliche, direkte Blutdruckmessungen im Alltag und beim Sport. Dtsch. med. Wschr. *95*, 741 (1970)
3. Badeer, H. S.: Contractile tension in the myocardium. Amer. Heart J. *66*, 432 (1963)
4. Bevegard, S., Holmgren, A., Jonnsson, B.: The effect of body position on the circulation at rest and during exercise, with special reference to the influence on the stroke volume. Acta physiol. scand. *49*, 279 (1960)
5. Bing, R. J.: The coronary circulation in health and disease as studied by sinus catheterization. Bull. N.Y. Acad. Med. *27*, 407 (1951)
6. Bock, K. D.: Medikamentöse Therapie der Hypertonie. In: Arterielle Hypertonie. Heintz, R., Losse, H. (eds.). p. 346. Stuttgart: Thieme 1969
7. Bohr, D. F.: Adrenergic receptors in the coronary arteries. Ann. N. Y. Acad. Sci. *139*, 799 (1967)
8. Bretschneider, H. J.: Aktuelle Probleme der Koronardurchblutung und des Myokardstoffwechsels. Regensburg ärztl. Fortbild. *1*, 11 (1967)
9. Bretschneider, H. J., Cott, L., Hilgert, C., Probst, R., Rau, G.: Gaschromatographische Trennung und Analyse von Argon als Basis einer neuen Fremdgasmethode zur Durchblutungsmessung von Organen. Verh. dtsch. Ges. Kreisl.-Forsch. *32*, 267 (1966)
10. Brod, J.: Die Nieren. Berlin: VEB Volk und Gesundheit 1964
11. Bürger, S., Meinardus, A., Strauer, B. E.: Hypertrophiegrad und Dynamik des linken Ventrikels bei der spontanen essentiellen Hypertonie der Ratte. Klin. Wschr. *56*, 207 (1978)
12. Bürger, S., Strauer, B. E.: Ventrikelfunktion und Kontraktilitätsreserve bei der spontanen essentiellen Hypertonie der Ratte. Verh. dtsch. Ges. Kreisl.-Forsch. *43*, 259 (1977)
13. Clawson, B. J.: The Heart in Essential Hypertension. Bell, E. T. (ed.). Minneapolis: Univ. Minnesota 1951
14. Cohn, J. N.: Blood pressure and cardiac performance. Amer. J. Med. *55*, 351 (1973)
15. Cohn, J. N., Rodriguera, E., Guiha, N. H.: Left ventricular function in hypertensive heart disease. In: Hypertension: Mechanisms and Management. Onesti, G., Kim, K. E., Moyer, J. H. (eds.), p. 191. New York: Grune und Stratton 1973
16. Cothran, L. N., Bowie, W. C., Hinds, J. E., Hawthorne, E. W.: Left ventricular wall thickness changes in unanesthetized horses. In: Factors Influencing Myocardial Contractility. Tanz, R. D., et al. (ed.), p. 163. New York: Academic Press 1967
17. Covell, J. W., Braunwald, E., Ross, J. jr., Sonnenblick, E. H.: Studies on digitalis. XVI. Effects on myocardial oxygen consumption. J. clin. Invest. *45*, 1535 (1966)
18. Daggett, W. M., Weisfeldt, M. L.: Influence of the sympathetic nervous system on the response of the normal heart to digitalis. Amer. J. Cardiol. *16*, 394 (1965)
19. DeMots, H., Rahimtoola, S. H., Kremkau, E. L., Bennett, W., Mahler, D.: Effects of ouabain on myocardial oxygen supply and demand in patients with chronic coronary artery disease. J. clin. Invest. *58*, 312 (1976)
20. Dumesnil, J. G., Ritman, E. L., Frye, R. L., Gau, G. T., Rutherford, B. D., Davis, G. D.: Quantitative determination of regional left ventricular wall dynamics by Roentgen videometry. Circulation *50*, 700 (1974)
21. Eber, L. M., Greenby, H. M., Cooke, J. M., Gorlin, R.: Dynamic changes in wall thickness of the human left ventricle. Circulation *36* (Suppl. II), 100 (1967)
22. Feigl, E. O., Fry, D. L.: Myocardial muscle thickness during the cardiac cycle. Circulat. Res. *14*, 451 (1964)

23. Ford, L. E.: Heart size. Circulat. Res. *39*, 297 (1976)

24. Frank, S., Braunwald, E.: Idiopathic hypertrophic subaortic stenosis. Clinical analysis of 126 patients with emphasis on the natural history. Circulation *37*, 759 (1968)

25. Frohlich, E.: Clinical-physiologic classification of hypertensive heart disease in essential hypertension. In: Hypertension: Mechanisms and Management. Onesti, G., Kim, K. E., Moyer, J. H. (eds.), p. 181. New York: Grune and Stratton 1973

26. Frohlich, E., Tarazi, R. C., Dustan, H. P.: Clinical-physiological correlations in the development of hypertensive heart diesease. Circulation *44*, 446 (1971)

27. Gaasch, W. H., Battle, W. E., Oboler, A. A., Banas, J. S., Levine, H. J.: Left ventricular stress and compliance in man. Circulation *45*, 746 (1972)

28. Gaasch, W. H., Levine, H. J., Quinones, M. A., Alexander, J. K.: Left ventricular compliance: mechanisms and clinical implications. Amer. J. Cardiol. *38*, 645 (1976)

29. Gaasch, W. H., Quinones, M. A., Weisser, E., Thiel, H. G., Alexander, J. K.: Diastolic compliance of the left ventricle in man. Amer. J. Cardiol. *36*, 193 (1975)

30. Gault, J. H., Ross, J., jr., Braunwald, E.: Contractile state of the left ventricle in man. Circulat. Res. *22*, 451 (1968)

31. Gillmann, H., Bernauer, K., Pankow, H.: Über die Fehlerbreite indirekter Blutdruckbestimmungen. Lebensversicherer.-Med. *20*, 111 (1968)

32. Gracey, D. R., Brandfonbremer, M.: The effect of lantoside C on coronary vascular resistance. Amer. Heart J. *66*, 88 (1963)

33. Grossman, W., McLaurin, L. P., Moos, S. P., Stefadouros, M., Young, D. T.: Wall thickness and diastolic properties of the left ventricle. Circulation *49*, 129 (1974)

34. Hansson, L., Aberg, H., Jameson, S., Karlberg, B., Malmcrona, R.: Initial clinical experience with J. C. I. 66,082, a new beta-adrenergic blocking agent, in hypertension. Acta med. scand. *194*, 549 (1973)

35. Harmjanz, D., Kochsiek, K., Heimburg, P., Emrich, J.: Auswirkungen der irregulär hypertrophischen Kardiomyopathie auf die Funktion und Form des rechten und linken Ventrikels. Z. Kreisl.-Forsch. *56*, 567 (1967)

36. Hawthorne, E.: Instantaneous dimensional changes of the left ventricle in dogs. Circulat. Res. *9*, 110 (1961)

37. Heintz, R.: Akute hypertensive Krisen bei essentieller und renaler Hypertonie. In: Aktuelle Hypertonieprobleme. Losse, H., Heintz, R. (eds.), p. 120. Stuttgart: Thieme 1973

38. Hood, W. P.: Dynamics of hypertrophy in left ventricular wall of man. In: Cardiac Hypertrophy. Alpert, N. R. (ed.), p. 445. New York: Academic Press 1971

39. Hood, W. P., Rackley, C. E., Rolett, E. L.: Wall stress in the normal and hypertrophied left ventricle. Amer. J. Cardiol. *22*, 550 (1968)

40. Hood, W. P., Thomson, W. J., Rackley, C. E., Rolett, E. L.: Comparison of calculation of left ventricular wall stress in man from thin-walled and thick-walled ellipsoidal models. Circul. Res. *24*, 575 (1969)

41. Hugenholtz, P. G., Kaplan, E., Hull, E.: Determination of left ventricular wall thickness by angiocardiography. Amer. Heart J. *78*, 513 (1969)

42. Jahnecke, J.: Die essentielle Hypertonie, ihre Beurteilung und die Grundsätze moderner Therapie. Ärztl. Fortbild. *18*, 206 (1970)

43. James, T.: Small arteries of the heart. Circulation *56*, 2 (1977)

44. Kannel, W. B., Dawber, T. R.: Hypertensive cardiovascular disease. The Framingham Study. In: Hypertension: Mechanisms and Management. Onesti, G., Kim, K. E., Moyer, J. H., (eds.), p. 93. New York: Grune and Stratton 1973

45. Kannel, W. B., Wolf, P. A., Verter, J., McNamara, P. M.: Epidemiologie assessment of the role of blood pressure in stroke. J. Amer. med. Ass. *214*, 301 (1970)

46. Kathke, N.: Die Veränderungen der Koronararterienzweige des Myokards bei Hypertonie. Beitr. path. Anat. *115*, 405 (1955)

47. Keith, N. M., Wagener, H. P., Barker, N. W.: Some different types of essential hypertension; their course and prognosis. Amer. J. med. Sci. *197*, 332 (1939)

48. Kennedy, J. W., Baxley, W. A., Figley, M. M., Dodge, H. T., Blackmon, J. R.: Quantitative angiocardiography: I. The normal left ventricle in man. Circulation *34*, 272 (1966)

49. Kochsiek, K., Heiss, H. W., Tauchert, M., Strauer, B. E.: Koronarreserve und Sauerstoffverbrauch bei hypertrophischer obstruktiver Cardiomyopathie. Verh. dtsch. Ges. inn. Med. *77*, 880 (1971)

50. Kochsiek, K., Larbig, D., Harmjanz, D.: Die hypertrophische obstruktive Kardiomyopathie.

Experiementelle Medizin, Pathologie und Klinik. Vol. 35, Berlin, Heidelberg, New York: Springer 1971

51. Kochsiek, T., Tauchert, M., Cott, L., Neubaur, J.: Die Koronarreserve bei Patienten mit Aortenvitien. Verh. dtsch. Ges. inn. Med. *76*, 214 (1970)

52. Kroenig, B.: Blutdruckvariabilität bei Hochdruckkranken. Heidelberg: Hüthig 1976

53. Lewis, P.: The essential action of propranolol in hypertension. Amer. J. Cardiol. *60*, 837 (1976)

54. Lichtlen, P., Baumann, P. C., Preter, B.: Zur selektiven Koronarographie: Klinisch-angiographische Analyse anhand von 250 Patienten. Arch. Kreisl.-Forsch. *59*, 287 (1969)

55. Limbourg, P., Just, H., Lang, K. F., Schölmerich, P.: Ventricular function at rest and during exercise in the hypertensive heart. In: Ventricular Function During Rest and Exercise. Roskamm, H., Hahn, C. (eds.). Berlin, Heidelberg, New York: Springer 1976

56. Linzbach, A. J.: Heart failure from the point of view of quantitative anatomy. Amer. J. Cardiol. *5*, 370 (1960)

57. Linzbach, A. J., Linzbach, M.: Die Herzdilatation. Klin. Wschr. *29*, 40 (1951)

58. Lochner, W.: Herz. In: Physiologie des Kreislaufes. Schütz, E. (eds.), Vol. I. Berlin, Heidelberg, New York: Springer 1971

59. Lund-Johansen, P.: Hemodynamics in early essential hypertension. Acta med. scand. *183*, Suppl. 482 (1967)

60. McKenna, D. H., Corliss, R. J., Sialer, S., Zarmstorff, W. C., Crumpton, W. C., Rowe, G. G.: Effect of propranolol on systemic and coronary hemodynamics at rest and during stimulated exercise. Circulat. Res. *19*, 520 (1966)

61. Meerson, F. S.: Hyperfunktion, Hypertrophie und Insuffizienz des Herzens. Berlin: VEB Volk und Gesundheit 1969

62. Mirsky, J.: Assessment of passive elastic stiffness of cardiac muscle: mathematical concepts, physiological and clinical consideration, directions of future research. Progr. cardiovasc. Dis. *28*, 277 (1976)

63. Mitchell, J. H., Wildenthal, K., Mullins, C. B.: Geometrical studies of the left ventricle utilizing biplane cinefluorography. Fed. Proc. *28*, 1334 (1969)

64. Nechwatal, W., König, E., Eversmann, A., Lehnert, J.: Zur Frage der Frühdigitalisierung bei Patienten mit arterieller Hypertonie. Dtsch. med. Wschr. *102*, 989 (1977)

65. Nechwatal, W., König, E., Eversmann, A., Saltner, K.: Untersuchungen zur Frage der Belastungsherzinsuffizienz bei Hypertonie. Z. Kardiol. *64*, 375 (1975)

66. Nechwatal, W., König, E., Kronski, D., Eversmann, H., Eversmann, T.: Hemodynamic response to digitalization in patients with hypertensive cardiovascular disease. Basic Res. Cardiol. *71*, 553 (1976)

67. Okamoto, K.: Spontaneous Hypertension. Berlin, Heidelberg, New York: Springer 1972

68. Onesti, G., Kim, K. E., Moyer, H. J.: Hypertension: Mechanisms and Management. New York: Grune and Stratton 1973

69. Page, L. B., Yager, H. M., Sidd, J. J.: Drugs in the management of hypertension. Amer. Heart J. *92*, 252 (1976)

70. Parratt, J. R.: Blockade of sympathetic beta-receptors in the myocardial circulation. Brit. J. Pharmacol. *24*, 601 (1965)

71. Peterson, K. L., Skloven, D., Ludbrook, P., Uther, J. B., Ross, J. jr.: Comparison of isovolumic and ejection phase indices of myocardial performance in man. Circulation *49*, 1088 (1974)

72. Philipp, T., Cordes, K., Distler, A.: Sympathikusaktivierbarkeit und blutdrucksenkende Wirkung einer Beta-Rezeptorenblockade bei essentieller Hypertonie. Dtsch. med. Wschr. *102*, 569 (1977)

73. Pickering, G. W.: High Blood Pressure. 2nd edition. London: Churchill 1968

74. Pitt, B., Elliot, E. C., Gregg, D. E.: Adrenergic receptor activity in the coronary arteries of the unaesthetized dog. Circulat. Res. *21*, 75 (1967)

75. Rackley, Ch. E., Dodge, H. T., Coble, Y. D., Hay, R. E.: A method for determining left ventricular mass in man. Circulation *29*, 666 (1964)

76. Rahn, K. H.: Sympathikoadrenales System und Hypertonie. In: Aktuelle Hypertonieprobleme. Losse, H., Heintz, R. (eds.), p. 55. Stuttgart: Thieme 1973

77. Ross, J. jr., Sonnenblick, E. H., Covell, J. W., Kaiser, C. A., Spiro, D.: The architecture of the heart in systole and diastole. Circulat. Res. *21*, 409 (1967)

78. Rowe, G. G., Castillo, C. A., Maxwell, G. M., Crumpton, C. W.: A hemodynamic study of hypertension including observations in coronary blood flow. Ann. intern. Med. *54*, 405 (1961)

79. Sandler, H.: Dimensional analysis of the heart – A review. Amer. J. med. Sci. *260*, 56 (1970)

80. Sandler, H., Dodge, H. T.: Left ventricular tension and stress in man. Circulat. Res. *13*, 91 (1963)
81. Sandler, H. Dodge, H. T.: The use of single plane angiocardiograms for the calculation of left ventricular volume in man. Amer. Heart J. *75*, 325 (1968)
82. Sannerstedt, R.: Hemodynamic response to exercise in patients with arterial hypertension. Acta med. scand. *180*, Suppl. 458 (1966)
83. Sarre, H.: Differentialdiagnose und Therapie des renalen Hochdrucks. Ärztl. Prax. *21*, 2201 (1969)
84. Schelbert, H. R., Kreuzer, H., Neuhaus, K. L., Spiller, P.: Die Bestimmung der lokalen Myokardfunktion aus dem Cineventrikulogramm bei Herzgesunden und Patienten mit koronarer Herzkrankheit. Klin. Wschr. *51*, 512 (1973)
85. Scherpe, A., Strauer, B. E.: Untersuchungen über die hämodynamischen Determinanten der Auswurffraktion des Herzens. Verh. dtsch. Ges. inn. Med. *82*, 1109 (1976)
86. Seldinger, S. I.: Catheter replacement of the needle in percutaneous arteriography. A new technique. Acta radiol. (Stockh.) *39*, 368 (1953)
87. Shand, D. G.: Drug therapy: propranolol. New. Engl. J. Med. *293*, 280 (1975)
88. Simon, H., Krayenbühl, H. P., Rutishauser, W., Preter, B.: The contractile state of the hypertrophied left ventricular myocardium in aortic stenosis. Amer. Heart J. *79*, 587 (1970)
89. Sokolow, M., Lyon, T.: The ventricular complex in left ventricular hypertrophy as obtained by unipolar precordial and limb leads. Amer. Heart J. *37*, 161 (1949)
90. Sonnenblick, E. H., Williams, J. F., Glick, G., Mason, D. T., Braunwald, E.: Studies on digitalis: XV. Effects of cardiac glycosides on myocardial force-velocity relations in the nonfailing human heart. Circulation *34*, 532 (1966)
91. Spann. J. F., Buccino, R. A., Sonnenblick, E. H., Braunwald, E.: Contractile state of cardiac muscle obtained from cats with experimentally produced ventricular hypertrophy and heart failure. Circulat. Res. *21*, 341 (1967)
92. Strauer, B. E.: Digitalis und Myokardinfarkt. Med. Klin. *48*, 1937 (1975)
93. Strauer, B. E.: Dynamik, Koronardurchblutung und Sauerstoffverbrauch des normalen und kranken Herzens. Basel: Karger 1975
94. Strauer, B. E.: Die hypertrophische obstruktive Kardiomyopathie. Internist *16*, 530 (1975)
95. Strauer, B. E.: Myocardial oxygen consumption in chronic heart disease: role of wall stress, hypertrophy and coronary reserve. Am. J. Med. *44*, 730 (1979)
96. Strauer, B. E.: Ventricular function and coronary hemodynamics in hypertensive heart disease. Am. J. Cardiol. *44*, 999 (1979)
97. Strauer, B. E.: Neuere Ergebnisse zur Pathophysiologie der Koronarinsuffizienz. Internist *18*, 294 (1977)
98. Strauer, B. E.: Die quantitative Bestimmung der Koronarreserve in der Diagnostik koronarer Durchblutungsstörungen. Internist *18*, 579 (1977)
99. Strauer, B. E., Beer, K., Heitlinger, K., Höfling, B.: Left ventricular systolic wall stress as a primary determinant of myocardial oxygen consumption: Comparative studies in patients with normal left ventricular function, with pressure and volume overload and with coronary heart disease. Basic Res. Cardiol. *72*, 306 (1977)
100. Strauer, B. E., Bolte, H.-D., Heimburg, P., Riecker, G.: Zur koronaren Herzkrankheit. II.: Eine Analyse diastolischer Druck-Volumen-Beziehungen und linksventrikulärer Dehnbarkeit an 110 Patienten. Z. Kardiol. *64*, 311 (1975)
101. Strauer, B. E., Brune, J., Schenk, H., Knoll, D., Perings, E.: Lupus cardiomyopathy. Cardiac mechanics, hemodynamics and coronary blood flow in uncomplicated systemic lupus erythematosus. Amer. Heart. J. *92*, 715 (1976)
102. Strauer, B. E., Heimburg, P., Riecker, G.: Spätdiastlische Druckanstiegsgeschwindigkeit und Dehnbarkeit des linken Ventrikels bei der koronaren Herzkrankheit. Verh. dtsch. Ges. Kreisl.-Forsch. *39*, 285 (1973)
103. Strauer, B. E., Kramer, H., Avenhaus, H., Bolte, H.-D., Lüderitz, B., Neubaur, J., Riecker, G.: Hämodynamik, Volumina und Dehnbarkeit des linken Ventrikels bei 167 Patienten mit angeborenen und erworbenen Herzfehlern. Klin. Wschr. *53*, 961 (1975)
104. Strauer, B. E., Kramer, H., Bolte, H.-D., Riecker, G.: Die Beziehungen zwischen Volumengrößen und Auswurffraktion des linken Ventrikels bei Mitral- und Aortenklappenregurgitation. Klin. Wschr. *53*, 975 (1975)
105. Strauer, B. E., Reploh, H. D., Cott, L., Tauchert, M., Bretschneider, H. J.: Koronar- und allgemeine

98

Kreislaufwirkungen von Octapressin (Phenylalanin^2-Lysin^8-Vasopressin) am narkotisierten intakten Hunde. Ärztl. Forsch. *23*, 227 (1969)

106. Strauer, B. E., Riecker, G.: Kontraktilitätsgrößen und linksventrikuläre Dehnbarkeit bei der koronaren Herzkrankheit. Verh. dtsch. Ges. inn. Med. *80*, 1069 (1974)

107. Strauer, B. E., Tauchert, M., Cott, L., Heiss, H. W., Kochsiek, K., Bretschneider, H. J.: Über den Einfluß verschiedener Größen der Herzmechanik auf den Sauerstoffverbrauch des suffizienten und insuffizienten linken Ventrikels bei Aortenvitien. Verh. dtsch. Ges. inn. Med. *77*, 876 (1971)

108. Strauer, B. E., Tauchert, M., Cott, L., Kochsiek, K., Bretschneider, H. J.: Simultane Bestimmung des Sauerstoffverbrauches und der Koronardurchblutung des linken Ventrikels bei Mitral- und Herzklappenfehlern mit einem neuen hämodynamischen Parameter und der Argon-Fremdgasmethode. Verh. dtsch. Ges. inn. Med. *76*, 217 (1970)

109. Strauer, B. E., Tauchert, M., Heiss, H. W., Kochsiek, K., Bretschneider, H. J.: On the relations between coronary blood flow, oxygen consumption and cardiac work in patients with and without angina pectoris. In: Myocardial Blood Flow in Man. Methods and Significance in Coronary Disease. Maseri, A. (ed.), pp. 465–475. Torino: Minerva Medica (on behalf of the I.S.C.) 1972

110. Stumpe, K. O., Kolloch, R., Vetter, H., Gramann, W., Krück, F., Ressel, Ch., Higuchi, W.: Acute and longterm studies of the mechanism of action of beta-blocking drugs in lowering blood pressure. Amer. J. Med. *60*, 853 (1976)

111. Tauchert, M.: Koronarreserve und maximaler Sauerstoffverbrauch des menschlichen Herzens. Basis Res. Cardiol. *68*, 183 (1973)

112. Varnauskas, E.: Studies in hypertensive cardiovascular disease with special reference to cardiac function. Scan. J. clin. Lab. Invest. 7, Suppl. 17 (1955)

113. Vatner, S. F., Higgins, C. B., Franklin, D., Braunwald, E.: Effects of digitalis glycoside on coronary and systemic dynamics in conscious dogs. Circulat. Res. *28*, 470 (1971)

114. Vaughn Williams, E. M., Raine, A. E. G., Cabrera, H. A., Whyte, J. M.: The effects of prolonged beta-adrenoreceptor blockade on heart size and cardiac intracellular potentials in rabbits. Cardiovasc. Res. *9*, 579 (1975)

115. Völker, W., Strauer, B. E., Riecker, G.: Die maximale Verkürzungsgeschwindigkeit (V60^{max}) am hypertrophierten linken Ventrikel des Meerschweinchens beim Goldblatt-Hochdruck. Verh. dtsch. Ges. Kreisl.-Forsch. *38*, 161 (1972)

116. Wallace, J. M.: Hemodynamic lesions in hypertension. Amer. J. Cardiol. *36*, 670 (1975)

117. Weiss, L., Lundgren, Y., Folkow, B.: Effects of prolonged treatment with adrenergic betareceptor antagonists on blood pressure, cardiovascular design and reactivity in spontaneously hypertensive rats (SHR). Acta physiol. scand. *91*, 447 (1974)

118. Whitsitt, L. S., Lucchesi, B. R.: Effects of propranolol and its stereoisomers upon coronary vascular resistance. Circulat. Res. *21*, 305 (1967)

119. Wigle, E. D., Felderhof, C. H., Silver, M. D., Adelman, A. G.: Hypertrophic obstructive cardiomyopathy. In: Myocardial Diseases (Ed. N. O. Fowler), pp. 297–318. New York: Grune and Stratton 1973

120. Wong, A. Y. K., Rautaharju, P. M.: Stress distribution within the left ventricular wall approximated as a thick ellipsoidal shell. Amer. Heart. J. *75*, 649 (1968)

121. World Heath Organisation: Hypertension and coronary heart disease: Classification and criteria for epidemiological studies. First report of the expert committee on cardiovascular diseases and hypertension. Techn. Rep. Ser. *168* (1959)

122. World Health Organisation: Arterial hypertension and ischemic heart disease, preventive aspects. Report of an expert committee. Techn. Rep. Ser. *231* (1962)

6 Subject Index

102